HEALTHY EATING AND LIFESTYLE CHOICES FOR TYPE 2 DIABETES

A Practical Guide to Managing Blood Sugar, Improving Energy, and Living Well

DR ENO OLUWOLE

Healthy Eating and Lifestyle Choices for Type 2 Diabetes
A Practical Guide to Managing Blood Sugar, Improving Energy, and Living Well
© 2025 Dr Eno Oluwole

Author's Disclaimer

This book draws on research, professional experience, and an understanding of the challenges faced by individuals living with type 2 diabetes and is intended for informational and educational purposes only. It is not a substitute for professional medical advice, diagnosis, or treatment. While every effort has been made to provide accurate and up-to-date information, health knowledge is continually evolving; readers should consult their healthcare professionals about any health-related concerns they may have.

Legal Disclaimer

Always seek the advice and guidance of your healthcare professional with any questions you may have regarding your health, medical condition, or before starting any new health, nutrition, exercise, or lifestyle programme. Never disregard your healthcare professional's medical advice or delay seeking it because of something you have read in this book.

The author and publisher accept no responsibility or liability for any direct, indirect, or consequential loss, injury, or damage claimed to result from the use of any information or suggestions in this book. Readers are responsible for their own health decisions and should consult their healthcare professionals for personalised advice suited to their individual circumstances.

ISBN (Paperback): 978-1-7385330-1-5
Published by Eno Oluwole (self-published through IngramSpark)
Print in the country where it is sold
Author's Website: www.drenooluwole.com

DEDICATION

This book is dedicated to everyone living with type 2 diabetes, those supporting loved ones, and anyone taking steps to prevent it.

ACKNOWLEDGEMENTS

This book was made possible through the support and inspiration of many people.

I thank my family for their love and support throughout this journey.

To my friends, thank you for your wisdom and faith in this work.

To those living with type 2 diabetes, your stories and determination inspired this book. Thank you.

To the healthcare professionals, researchers, and educators whose expertise and dedication to evidence-based care have shaped the guidance you will find here, I am grateful for your commitment to health and well-being.

To you, the reader, I express my gratitude for allowing me to be part of your journey toward better health. May these pages provide the knowledge, hope, and confidence you need to live your healthiest life.

Above all, I thank God for the grace, strength, and purpose that made this book possible.

CONTENTS

PREFACE

Managing type 2 diabetes is a journey that goes far beyond blood sugar readings and medication schedules. It requires understanding your body, making informed decisions, and cultivating habits for long-term health. I wrote this book to offer practical guidance that empowers readers to adopt changes that can transform their quality of life.

Over the years, I have witnessed how knowledge replaces uncertainty with confidence. This book combines evidence-based strategies and first-hand insights, covering nutrition, exercise, stress management, and more, to help individuals effectively manage or reduce their risk of developing type 2 diabetes.

My goal is to make complex medical information accessible and understandable, without compromising the scientific accuracy it deserves, while also offering a practical, supportive, and judgment-free approach tailored to real-life challenges. Unlike general guides, this book combines evidence-based medical strategies with deep insights and actionable steps to help you navigate your journey with confidence.

Whether you are newly diagnosed, supporting someone, or looking to prevent type 2 diabetes, I hope this book offers the knowledge and strategies you need to manage blood sugar, improve energy, and thrive.

- Dr Eno Oluwole

INTRODUCTION

When Sue entered her doctor's office, she thought she was only there for a routine check-up. She had been feeling more tired than usual and experiencing increased thirst. She had also noticed that she was visiting the bathroom more often, but had attributed it to stress and a busy work schedule.

After a few blood tests, she heard the words she was not expecting: "You have type 2 diabetes."

Sue's first reaction was fear, quickly replaced by confusion. Her mind filled with questions. What did this mean for her future? Would her diet have to change? As she sat in the doctor's office, the weight of the diagnosis began to settle in. Determined not to let it define her, Sue took control of her health. She decided to understand type 2 diabetes and investigate research-backed lifestyle choices for effective management. She knew support from loved ones would help, and working with her doctor would offer essential guidance.

Motivated to take control, Sue explored evidence-based healthy eating pattern, attended the diabetes educational programme, and connected with others on a similar journey. She discovered that type 2 diabetes is a lifestyle-related condition that can be prevented, managed, or even put into remission through healthy dietary and lifestyle choices. Sue learned that progress comes from making small, consistent changes every day, rather than striving for perfection. As she integrated new habits, she noticed her energy and mood improved, which motivated her to stay committed. Inspired by her progress, Sue started a blog to encourage others to embrace healthy habits and build a supportive community.

This book explains type 2 diabetes and offers a unique blend of practical, evidence-based guidance, supportive strategies, and real-world solutions for making lasting changes. You will discover how targeted, actionable decisions about food and lifestyle can help you regain energy and improve your health.

Whether you are newly diagnosed with type 2 diabetes like Sue, have been managing it for years, aim to achieve remission, or wish to prevent it, this book is uniquely designed to give you practical, straightforward, and evidence-based guidance. You will find support, encouragement, and clarity in every chapter as you learn how food choices, physical activity, stress management, daily habits, and, if needed, medication work together to support your blood sugar, energy, and overall well-being.

Within these pages, you will find:

- How to build a diabetic-friendly plate that maintains steady blood sugar levels without feeling deprived
- Easy ways to integrate physical activity into your daily routine
- How stress and sleep affect blood sugar, and what you can do about it
- Why collaborating with your healthcare team can make all the difference
- Practical strategies for maintaining motivation, even when life becomes hectic or challenging

Type 2 diabetes does not define you. With the correct information, practical tools, consistent strategies, and support, you can reduce blood sugar swings, improve your energy, and focus on prevention, control, or even remission—empowering you to live a healthier life.

Let us get started, one step, one meal, and one choice at a time.

PART

I

UNDERSTANDING TYPE 2 DIABETES

CHAPTER 1
DIABETES OVERVIEW & EPIDEMIOLOGY

Type 2 diabetes was rare until the 19th century. In 2024, 589 million adults (20-79 years) were living with diabetes worldwide, and the numbers are rising[1]. Type 2 diabetes is estimated to affect one in nine adults, making it a significant concern for everyone. Friends or family may also be affected. Poor dietary choices and the consumption of ultra-processed foods, which are high in sugars and unhealthy fats, have contributed to this global problem (Willett, 2001).

Global Diabetes Prevalence Data by Region–2024 (International Diabetes Federation Data):

- North America and the Caribbean: 56 million

- South and Central America: 35 million

- Europe: 66 million

- Africa: 25 million

- Middle East and North Africa: 85 million

- South-East Asia: 107 million

- Western Pacific: 215 million

These figures do not tell the whole story. According to the International Diabetes Federation, over 40% of people with diabetes are unaware they have the condition, and three-quarters of cases among adults occur in low- and middle-income countries. This global trend is largely driven by the increasing adoption of unhealthy diets, sedentary lifestyles, and environmental factors in those regions.

In many regions, type 2 diabetes is more prevalent in urban areas than in rural ones, primarily due to differences in physical activity, diet, and lifestyle. However, in high-income countries such as the UK and much of Europe, the urban–rural gap is less noticeable.

The rise in type 2 diabetes is closely linked to obesity, making the condition more common in nations with high obesity rates (Menke, 2014). This pattern is evident in affluent regions, including the United States, Western Europe, and parts of the Middle East. However, type 2 diabetes is no longer confined to wealthier countries. As economic development expands in other parts of the world, so too do obesity, calorie-dense diets, and sedentary lifestyles, all of which drive the growing global burden of the disease.

Diabetes is not a modern disease. The ancient Egyptians, Greeks, and Indians all recognised it and described it. They also understood the different types.

What is new, however, is the global scale of the diabetes epidemic. An article in Diabetes Research and Clinical Practice describes it as 'a pandemic of unprecedented magnitude', now affecting roughly one in 10 adults worldwide[2]. Unlike other pandemics, this one is mainly driven by lifestyle choices, which means we have the power to change its course by adopting healthier habits. Type 2 diabetes is preventable, and by making informed decisions about our diet and lifestyle, we can significantly reduce our risk, offering hope for a healthier future.

Over the past hundred years, significant lifestyle changes have led to the rise in obesity and type 2 diabetes. Until the 19th century, obesity was rare. Most people did physical labour from dawn to dusk, slept longer hours, and lived in tune with the natural cycles of sunlight.

Today, the situation is quite different. Food is abundant, and calorie intake often exceeds what the body can burn. Daily life has become more sedentary, characterised by decreased physical activity, shorter sleep durations, and increased screen and gadget use. These wide-ranging changes have led to the twin epidemics of obesity and diabetes. To reverse the trend, lifestyle changes must be as significant as those that caused the problem.

What is diabetes, and what is type 2 diabetes?

Many people think of diabetes as just one condition, but this is not correct. There are different types, each with its own cause and challenges.

Classification of Diabetes Mellitus[3]

Diabetes mellitus includes several distinct types, each characterised by specific causes and clinical features. The main categories relevant to clinical practice are type 1 diabetes, type 2 diabetes, gestational diabetes, and a few less common forms caused by other factors. Clearly distinguishing these categories is essential for understanding disease mechanisms, assessing risk, and guiding management.

1. **Type 1 diabetes**: This accounts for about 5–10% of all diabetes cases worldwide and is the most common form of diabetes in children and young people (BMJ Best Practice, n.d.). It is an autoimmune disease characterised by the destruction of insulin-producing beta cells in the pancreas.

2. **Type 2 Diabetes:** This is the most common type, affecting over 90% of adults living with the condition. (McKeever Bullard,

2018). It is a lifestyle-related condition, and as it is the most common type, this book will primarily focus on it and how to prevent, manage, and effectively put it into remission.

3. **Gestational diabetes**: This type of diabetes is first diagnosed at or after 24 weeks of pregnancy. Many women diagnosed with gestational diabetes (GDM) have a substantially higher risk of developing type 2 diabetes later in life (Bellamy, Casas, Hingorani, & Williams, 2009).

4. **Other types of diabetes** may be caused by damage to the pancreas resulting from medications, substances, toxins, or other autoimmune conditions.

Type 2 diabetes is a long-term condition where the body either does not produce enough insulin or the insulin it produces does not work effectively, a state known as insulin resistance (Cleveland Clinic, 2025). This impaired insulin function results in elevated blood sugar levels, which, if not properly managed, can lead to a range of serious health complications (American Diabetes Association, 2023). Evidence also shows that poorly controlled type 2 diabetes is associated with a reduced life expectancy, emphasising the importance of early diagnosis and effective management (Livingston et al., 2023).

Type 2 diabetes affects more than just blood sugar. Over time, it interferes with the metabolism of fats, proteins, vitamins, and minerals. Many people with type 2 diabetes also suffer from high levels of 'bad' cholesterol, slower healing, and various nutritional deficiencies. More seriously, type 2 diabetes can lead to heart disease, kidney disease, and nerve damage. (Diabetes UK, n.d.; NHS, n.d.).

How does type 2 diabetes develop?

Contrary to popular belief, type 2 diabetes does not begin with insulin deficiency. In its early stages, the body produces more insulin to try to manage rising glucose levels. Type 2 diabetes is mainly associated with obesity caused by excessive calorie consumption, although genetic factors can also influence its development (McCarthy, 2001; Li et al., 2011). When people consume more calories than they need, the surplus is stored as fat, increasing the risk of obesity and other metabolic disorders. It is important to recognise that having a genetic predisposition does not guarantee the development of diabetes, highlighting that the condition can often be prevented through healthy eating, regular physical activity, and other lifestyle strategies, as we will discuss.

When we consume too many calories, blood glucose levels rise. Carbohydrates are the primary source of this glucose, but the liver can also produce glucose by converting amino acids from protein and, to a lesser extent, glycerol from fats (Felig, 1977). Glucose itself is not harmful; it is the body's preferred energy source, fuelling muscles, the brain, and other organs. The issue, however, arises when there is an excessive amount of glucose in the bloodstream.

Insulin, produced by the beta cells in the pancreas, plays a central role in this process. Acting like a key, it signals to the muscles, liver, and other tissues to absorb glucose effectively, 'unlocking' cells for energy use. When calorie intake exceeds the body's needs, the pancreas produces extra insulin to keep glucose under control. Over time, this can result in two significant issues: insulin resistance and beta-cell stress and decline.

1. Insulin resistance occurs when body tissues gradually become less sensitive to insulin, impairing its signals and diminishing the body's ability to utilise glucose for energy. This explains why many people with type 2 diabetes experience fatigue and other symptoms.

2. Beta cell stress and decline. The insulin-producing cells in the pancreas, over time, become overworked and may eventually fail, leading to relative insulin deficiency. At this stage, diabetes can be said to result from both insulin resistance and reduced insulin production.

Chronic high blood glucose levels damage the body in multiple ways. It disrupts fluid balance, harms cells, and causes dehydration, which explains the excessive thirst often experienced by people with diabetes. Impaired insulin function also slows tissue repair, contributing to damage in nerves, blood vessels, and organs.

Other organs attempt to compensate but also suffer over time. The liver, which helps regulate blood glucose, may become inflamed and store fat. The kidneys filter excess glucose into urine, resulting in frequent urination. Prolonged stress on the kidneys makes diabetes a leading cause of kidney disease and kidney failure in the UK and worldwide (Diabetes UK, n.d.; Kidney Research UK, 2024).

In summary, type 2 diabetes typically begins with excessive calorie intake, resulting in elevated blood glucose levels, which in turn lead to increased insulin production, beta cell strain, and ultimately, insulin resistance. This results in higher blood glucose and progressive organ damage. Understanding this process underscores the importance of adopting healthy eating habits and making lifestyle changes to both prevent and manage the condition.

A Step-by-Step Explanation

1. Excess calorie intake
   - Consuming more calories than the body requires, especially from refined carbohydrates and fats, results in weight gain and increased fat storage.

2. Rising blood glucose levels
   - Carbohydrates are broken down into glucose, which is the body's main fuel. When consumed excessively, blood glucose levels rise above normal.

3. Improved insulin production
   - The pancreas responds by producing more insulin, the hormone that facilitates the movement of glucose into cells for energy or storage.

4. Insulin resistance begins

   - Over time, the body's tissues (muscles, liver, and fat cells) become less responsive to insulin. Cells stop 'listening' to insulin's signal, making it more difficult for glucose to enter.

5. Beta cell stress

   - To compensate, the pancreas works harder and produces even more insulin. This constant demand stresses the insulin-producing beta cells.

6. Beta cell decline

   - Eventually, these cells become exhausted, and their capacity to produce insulin decreases. At this point, the body experiences both insulin resistance and a relative insulin deficiency.

7. Persistent high blood glucose levels

   - With decreased insulin effectiveness, glucose builds up in the blood. Long-term hyperglycaemia harms blood vessels, nerves, kidneys, and other organs.

8. Complications arise

   - Untreated or poorly controlled type 2 diabetes can cause long-term problems such as heart disease, kidney disease, nerve damage, vision issues, slow wound healing, and a higher risk of early death.

However, it is important to note that certain complications, such as nerve pain and eye changes, often improve with better blood sugar control within a few months of intensive diabetes management (The Diabetes Control and Complications Trial Research Group, 1993).

Diabetes Risk Factors, Signs, Symptoms, and Diagnosis

Before proceeding, let us quickly review the risk factors for diabetes, its symptoms, and some standard diagnostic tests.

Risk Factors

When it comes to risk factors, excessive calorie intake and low-calorie expenditure leading to obesity are the leading causes of type 2 diabetes. (Excess calorie intake is more likely to cause obesity than lack of exercise, Diabetes.co.uk, 2025).

Other risk factors include:

- Advanced age
- Physical inactivity
- Family history of diabetes, and
- Certain ethnicities, such as South Asian, African, or Hispanic backgrounds

Additional risk factors include a history of:

- Gestational diabetes
- Polycystic ovary syndrome.
- Hypertension
- Dyslipidaemia
- And cardiovascular disease

Signs and Symptoms

Type 2 diabetes often develops gradually and may be asymptomatic for many years. When symptoms occur, they usually include:

- Increased thirst (polydipsia)
- Frequent urination (polyuria)
- Increased hunger (polyphagia)

These are called the 3Ps of diabetes.

Furthermore:

- Unexplained weight loss
- Fatigue
- Blurred vision
- Slow-healing wounds
- Recurrent infections

Remember that, especially in the initial stages of diabetes, symptoms tend to be subtle and nonspecific, such as:

- Fatigue
- Excessive sweating
- And other minor issues

Therefore, it is not uncommon for diabetes to be diagnosed during a routine checkup for another health condition.

Diagnosis

Diagnosing type 2 diabetes usually involves blood tests to measure blood glucose levels. Common tests include:

- Fasting Blood Sugar Test: This assesses blood sugar levels following an overnight fast.
- Oral Glucose Tolerance Test (OGTT): After fasting, the patient consumes a glucose solution, and their blood sugar levels are subsequently measured.
- Haemoglobin A1c Test: This reflects the average blood glucose levels over the past two to three months.

These three major tests — Fasting Plasma Glucose (FPG), Oral Glucose Tolerance Test (OGTT), and Haemoglobin A1c (HbA1c) — help doctors in diagnosing type 2 diabetes and prediabetes.

Diagnostic Criteria for Diabetes and Prediabetes -American Diabetes Association (ADA)

Fasting Plasma Glucose (FPG)

- Normal: < 100 mg/dL (< 5.6 mmol/L)
- Prediabetes: 100–125 mg/dL (5.6–6.9 mmol/L)
- Diabetes: ≥ 126 mg/dL (≥ 7.0 mmol/L)

2-hour OGTT (75 g glucose)

- Normal: < 140 mg/dL (< 7.8 mmol/L)
- Prediabetes: 140–199 mg/dL (7.8–11.0 mmol/L)
- Diabetes: ≥ 200 mg/dL (≥ 11.1 mmol/L)

Haemoglobin A1c (HbA1c)

- Normal: < 5.7% (< 42 mmol/L)
- Prediabetes: 5.7–6.4% (42–47 mmol/L)
- Diabetes: ≥ 6.5% (≥ 48 mmol/L)

Note:

- **Prediabetes:** This is a broad term for blood glucose levels that are higher than normal but not high enough to diagnose type 2 diabetes. It is sometimes also known as impaired fasting glucose (IFG) or impaired glucose tolerance (IGT), depending on the specific blood test employed.
- **Type 2 Diabetes:** A single abnormal result for type 2 diabetes should be confirmed by repeat testing, except in cases of clear hyperglycaemia and classic symptoms.

Type 2 diabetes often develops quietly over time, and its signs and symptoms can sometimes go unnoticed until significant damage has occurred. Early detection is crucial for effective management and intervention.

Here are some common signs and symptoms to look out for:

- Increased thirst: Persistent thirst, often accompanied by dry mouth, can indicate high blood glucose levels.

- Frequent urination: As the kidneys work to excrete excess glucose, this can result in increased urination, particularly during the night.

- Fatigue: Feeling unusually tired or exhausted can result from the body's inability to utilise glucose for energy effectively.

- Blurred vision: High blood sugar levels can cause swelling in the eye lenses, leading to blurred vision.

- Slow-healing sores or Frequent infections: People may experience cuts or sores that take longer to heal, and they may have a heightened susceptibility to infections.

- Unexplained weight loss: Despite eating normally, some individuals may experience sudden weight loss because the body burns muscle and fat for energy when it cannot access glucose.

- Tingling or numbness: Nerve damage caused by prolonged high blood sugar levels can result in tingling, numbness, or pain in the hands and feet, a condition known as diabetic neuropathy.

- Dark patches on skin: Acanthosis nigricans, characterised by dark, velvety patches in body folds, can be a sign of insulin resistance.

If you notice any of these symptoms, it is crucial to consult a healthcare professional for evaluation. Early diagnosis and intervention can significantly improve outcomes and help prevent complications associated with diabetes.

By recognising the risk factors and being aware of the signs and symptoms, individuals can take steps to maintain their health and prevent the development of type 2 diabetes.

Of the diagnostic tests already discussed, fasting plasma glucose (FPG) remains the most commonly used test for diagnosing type 2 diabetes, mainly because it is simple, quick, inexpensive, and accessible even in resource-limited settings. For this test, a person should ideally have their blood drawn after fasting for 8 hours but no more than 12 hours, as fasting periods longer than this can produce false results. Extended fasting naturally results in lower blood glucose levels, which can be misleading. Likewise, if one has not fasted for enough time (less than 8 hours), it may cause unusually high blood glucose levels.

High-income countries, such as the UK, and major healthcare systems are increasingly adopting HbA1c as the primary diagnostic tool because it does not require fasting and reflects long-term blood sugar management. It is also an excellent test for individuals living with diabetes, as it indicates the average blood sugar level over the past three months. This is because this specific test measures glucose accumulated in red blood cells, which typically have an average lifespan of 90-120 days.

Sometimes, fasting plasma glucose (FPG) levels may appear normal due to prolonged fasting and dietary measures taken by patients before blood tests, which can conceal the actual values. However, HbA1c offers a more precise assessment in such cases. It reflects how well an individual has managed their blood glucose over the past two to three months.

Before we continue with our discussion, let us take a moment to discuss prediabetes further.

Prediabetes

This is not diabetes. It indicates a higher risk of developing it and suggests the need for urgent lifestyle modifications.

At this stage, medication is seldom required, although some doctors may occasionally consider it. Lifestyle changes and weight loss, if overweight or obese, are crucial in preventing the onset of diabetes. Prediabetes acts like an amber light–warning people early enough.

Why do early interventions matter?

Earlier, we discussed how type 2 diabetes develops, starting with excess calorie intake and progressing through stages that lead to insulin resistance, followed by reduced insulin production caused by stress and a decline in the number of insulin-producing beta cells in the pancreas. In its final stage, the disease results in damage to various organs.

As one might expect, reversing insulin resistance through lifestyle interventions is indeed possible. Therefore, if one begins early enough, before the nerves, blood vessels, liver, and kidneys sustain significant damage, putting type 2 diabetes into remission through lifestyle changes becomes considerably easier.

We do not suggest that lifestyle changes cease to be effective in advanced diabetes; they can still play a vital role. Healthy eating and regular exercise improve the body's ability to use insulin and help regulate blood sugar levels (Jiang et al., 2019; Stanford et al., 2022). They also reduce fat in the liver, which improves fatty liver disease (Promrat et al., 2010; Cusi, 2021; Keating et al., 2012), and they support other organs in functioning more effectively.

However, in more advanced stages of the disease, it becomes harder to repair damage fully, such as extensive loss of insulin-producing cells, significant kidney impairment, or nerve damage. Even so, lifestyle changes remain important in slowing further progression (Knowler et al., 2002; Holeček, 2025).

To put type 2 diabetes into remission, it is essential to begin integrating healthy eating and lifestyle changes into your daily routine as early as possible.

CHAPTER 2
THE ROLE OF LIFESTYLE IN MANAGING DIABETES

You may wonder why healthcare professionals emphasise lifestyle changes so much when medications are available. When asked how they manage their diabetes, many people respond, 'I take my medications.' While it is true that medication helps, it does not address the root cause of diabetes. Instead, it merely controls some effects of an unhealthy lifestyle. Therefore, even if you take your medications daily, the condition can still worsen over time if you do not adapt your lifestyle.

Taking medications can slow the progression of diabetes, but on their own, they are not sufficient. For a lifestyle-related condition such as type 2 diabetes, lifestyle interventions are crucial.

Medications like metformin can help reduce insulin resistance and support some weight loss. Newer options, such as Ozempic, can lead to even greater weight reduction. However, these changes do not happen naturally, and there are concerns about drug side effects. The good news is that lifestyle modifications, such as adopting healthier eating habits, engaging in regular physical activity, stress management, and other lifestyle strategies, work in harmony with your body. Unlike medications, these approaches can address the root cause of the problem and offer long-term health benefits.

Some diabetes medications, such as sulfonylureas, work by stimulating the pancreas to produce more insulin, effectively lowering blood sugar levels. There is, however, mixed evidence on the long-term effects on β-cell function. For this reason, people taking these medications should be regularly monitored by their healthcare professionals to ensure they remain safe and effective for long-term diabetes management.

There are also medications known to reduce the risk of heart and kidney disease. Remember, however, that they are not a replacement for lifestyle changes.

We are not suggesting that people stop treatment. Instead, we recommend that individuals recognise that medication is not a substitute for adopting healthy eating and lifestyle interventions. Furthermore, lifestyle changes offer greater and more lasting health benefits.

Below are some oral medications commonly used to manage type 2 diabetes. They are valuable and helpful, but they are just beneficial tools [4].

Common Diabetes Medications and What They Do

Biguanides: These are a class of medications that includes metformin. They help the body use insulin more effectively and reduce the amount of sugar the liver produces. They rarely cause weight gain, and they may even help you lose some weight. They usually do not cause hypoglycaemia.

Sulfonylureas (such as Glimepiride and gliclazide): These medications stimulate the pancreas to produce more insulin, which helps lower blood sugar levels.

DPP-4 inhibitors (such as sitagliptin and linagliptin): These prolong the action of certain natural hormones. When blood sugar levels are high, these hormones signal the body to release insulin. These medications rarely affect your weight and seldom cause low blood sugar.

SGLT2 inhibitors (such as empagliflozin and dapagliflozin): These help the kidneys eliminate excess sugar from the body through urine. They can help lower blood sugar, aid in weight loss, reduce blood pressure, and protect the heart.

GLP-1 receptor agonists (such as Liraglutide and Semaglutide): These medications mimic a natural hormone, prompting the body to release more insulin when blood sugar levels are high and reducing glucagon, another hormone that raises blood sugar levels. They are beneficial for heart health, promote weight loss, and have a low risk of hypoglycaemia.

Thiazolidinediones (such as pioglitazone): They make muscle and fat cells more responsive to insulin. They reduce blood sugar levels, liver fat, and liver inflammation, leading to improved fatty liver disease.

Evidence-based lifestyle interventions

In the section 'How diabetes develops?' we discussed that diabetes begins with 'excessive calorie intake and low-calorie expenditure,' leading to obesity, as the root cause of the disease. However, it is not just about calories. Ultra-processed foods, rich in refined carbohydrates and industrial oils, significantly contribute to hormonal imbalances that increase hunger and promote insulin resistance (Ludwig, 2016). Keep this in mind. To explain, consider how a drive-thru breakfast of a bacon, egg, and cheese sandwich with hash browns and a sugary latte compares to a whole-food breakfast of oatmeal topped with berries and a handful of almonds, accompanied by herbal tea. The whole-food choice provides steady, sustained energy and nutrients without the blood sugar spike and the risk of insulin resistance associated with the ultra-processed alternative.

Nutrition therapy, dietary adjustments, and physical activity are essential components of any diabetes management plan, regardless of the stage or severity of the disease. These measures must be implemented and adhered to carefully, as numerous clinical studies have affirmed their effectiveness.

Before we proceed, let us discuss one of the most important questions: How much can someone benefit from lifestyle interventions, and what clinical evidence supports them?

DiRECT – Clinical Study That Changed How We View Diabetes.

For years, healthcare professionals denied that diabetes could go into remission. However, everything changed with the **DiRECT** clinical study. It marked a significant shift and brought an end to years of controversy. Ultimately, it confirmed that lifestyle changes can lead to remission of type 2 diabetes in many cases. Healthcare professionals have since then agreed that diabetes 'remission' is possible even without medications.

The DiRECT study is a landmark clinical trial conducted in the UK that involved individuals with mild to moderate diabetes who had preserved insulin production. Participants were aged 20-65 years with type 2 diabetes of less than 6 years duration, and a BMI of 27-45 kg/m2, who were not receiving insulin.

The study lasted between 12 and 20 weeks. Participants in the intervention group followed a structured weight management programme that started with a low-calorie diet (approximately 800 kcal/day) supplemented with replacements, such as shakes and soups. They then gradually reintroduced foods into their diets and received ongoing support to help them sustain the weight loss.

The aim was to lose enough weight and keep it off to reverse the underlying causes of type 2 diabetes. The study followed them for two and then five years.

After two years, the intervention resulted in complete remission of type 2 diabetes in 36% of participants. By five years, 13% remained in remission, free of the condition and not requiring any diabetes medications (DiRECT Study, 2024) [5].

The study provided strong evidence that intensive weight management can lead to remission of type 2 diabetes, even in individuals with moderately severe disease and preserved insulin production.

So, what is stopping you? The clinical evidence is available. Ultimately, it is your choice whether to make these lifestyle changes or not.

What about the Diabetes Prevention Programme (DPP)?

In the landmark **DPP trial,** intensive lifestyle interventions, including modest dietary changes, regular exercise, and a 5–10% reduction in body weight, reduced the incidence of type 2 diabetes by approximately 58%, compared to 31% with metformin in high-risk individuals [6].

While metformin remains a first-line therapy for managing type 2 diabetes, multiple trials (Knowler et al., 2002; Tuomilehto et al., 2001; Li et al., 2008) have shown that lifestyle changes can be more effective for prevention. The DPP found that lifestyle modification was nearly twice as effective as metformin in delaying or preventing the onset of diabetes.

However, long-term follow-ups suggest that the differences diminish over time, so continued commitment to lifestyle changes remains crucial for achieving lasting benefits.

Hopefully, the findings from the two studies discussed demonstrate that lifestyle interventions are crucial for individuals seeking to prevent and manage diabetes.

In the following chapters, we will explore in more detail how to implement strategies for lifestyle interventions that can help individuals overcome diabetes. Here is a list of some of the most effective lifestyle interventions:

1. **Medical Nutrition Therapy**

   Individualised meal planning is a key strategy for diabetes management. It involves tailoring your diet to your specific needs, with a focus on reducing total caloric intake (if overweight), limiting refined carbohydrates, increasing dietary fibre, and emphasising whole grains, vegetables, legumes, and lean proteins.

2. **Regular Physical Activity**

   Engaging in at least 150 minutes of moderate-intensity aerobic exercise per week (e.g., brisk walking, cycling) combined with resistance training at least twice a week.

3. **Weight Loss**

   Achieving and maintaining a 5–10% reduction in initial body weight significantly improves glycaemic control and cardiovascular risk factors.

4. **Smoking Cessation**

   Quitting smoking reduces cardiovascular and microvascular complications and improves overall health outcomes.

5. **Limiting Alcohol Intake**

   Keeping alcohol consumption to recommended limits or stopping altogether, as we will explain later in 'Chapter 9', helps prevent negative effects on blood glucose and overall health.

6. **Behavioural Support**

Structured diabetes self-management education and ongoing behavioural counselling improve adherence to diet, exercise, and medication regimens.

7. **Adequate Sleep**

Maintaining regular sleep patterns and addressing sleep disorders is important, as poor sleep is associated with worse glycaemic control.

8. **Stress Management**

Incorporating mindfulness, relaxation techniques, or cognitive-behavioural strategies can help reduce stress, which can negatively impact blood glucose levels.

Common myths and misconceptions

Many misconceptions about type 2 diabetes still exist, often leading to misunderstanding or stigma. Addressing these myths is essential for effective diabetes prevention and management.

1. **Myth:** Eating sugar directly causes diabetes.

   Fact: Consuming sugar alone does not cause type 2 diabetes. The major contributors are excess calories resulting in overweight or obesity, as well as physical inactivity. A diet high in added sugars can also contribute to weight gain. Sugar provides rapidly absorbed carbohydrates, resulting in faster and larger glucose spikes, which can contribute to the development of insulin resistance.

2. **Myth:** People with diabetes must avoid all carbohydrates.

   Fact: Carbohydrates are an essential part of a balanced diet. The focus should be on portion control and choosing complex, high-fibre carbohydrates, rather than eliminating them.

3. **Myth**: Type 2 diabetes is not a severe disease.

   Fact: Type 2 diabetes can lead to serious complications, including heart disease, kidney failure, nerve damage, and vision loss, if not appropriately managed. It is now among the leading causes of death globally.

4. **Myth:** Natural remedies can cure diabetes.

   Fact: There is no scientific evidence that supplements, herbal remedies, or alternative therapies can cure diabetes. Evidence-based medical management and lifestyle modifications are essential for control.

5. **Myth:** People with diabetes cannot live everyday lives.

   Fact: With proper management, including diet, exercise, monitoring, and medication, most people with type 2 diabetes can lead healthy lives.

Therefore, dispelling these myths is essential for fostering understanding, lowering stigma, and promoting proper care for individuals with type 2 diabetes.

PART

II

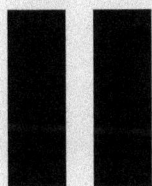

HEALTHY EATING FOR BLOOD SUGAR CONTROL

CHAPTER 3
FOOD AS MEDICINE

Food supplies us with energy or calories, structural materials, and more. It is also a source of vitamins, minerals, bioactive compounds, and specific signalling molecules, among other nutrients.

An unbalanced diet, characterised by an excess of certain nutrients, can be harmful to health. A diet high in rapidly absorbed carbohydrates and calories may cause problems such as obesity and diabetes.

However, these issues do not occur in a day or two; instead, they appear after prolonged neglect, resulting from years of consuming an unbalanced and unhealthy diet.

Humans need carbohydrates for energy. Fats also supply energy and help form body structures, such as cell walls and hormones. Proteins, although they can be used as an energy source, are primarily used to build body structures.

An ideal diet includes all the macronutrients (carbohydrates, fats, and proteins) in balanced amounts, together with micronutrients such as vitamins and minerals.

When selecting an appropriate diet for managing diabetes, it is essential to consider several key factors, including total caloric intake, the specific types and proportions of carbohydrates and fats consumed, and, most importantly, the quality and quantity of carbohydrates included in the dietary pattern.

Before we proceed with carbohydrates, remember that choosing **fats** wisely is also crucial. Try to get about one-third of your calories from fat. Monounsaturated fats, found in olive oil, avocados, and certain nuts, are beneficial. Eating polyunsaturated fats in moderation, as part of a balanced omega-6 to omega-3 ratio, can also help. You should limit or avoid saturated fats, which are present in animal fats, palm oil, and coconut oil. Remember that one gram of fat contains more than twice the calories of one gram of carbohydrate or protein, so even a small amount of fat adds significantly to your overall energy intake.

When it comes to **protein**, consuming adequate amounts can enhance anabolic processes and help control appetite. A diet rich in high-quality protein, particularly from plant sources, fish, and lean meats, can be beneficial for people with diabetes, especially when paired with a balanced intake of carbohydrates and healthy fats. However, individuals with kidney disease, which is common in diabetes, should consult their healthcare professional before increasing protein intake, as excessive protein intake can damage the kidneys.

In this book, the main focus will be on carbohydrates; however, it is vital to understand that a balanced diet must contain a variety of nutrients.

Now, regarding **carbohydrates**, the rule is simple. Avoid eating them in large amounts, as they can lead to obesity and insulin resistance. Carbohydrates increase blood glucose levels more quickly than other macronutrients.

However, when choosing them, opt for complex carbohydrates, such as whole grains, instead of simple carbohydrates. Complex carbohydrates have larger molecules, which means they digest more slowly, resulting in a gradual rise in blood glucose levels. Simple carbohydrates, such as sugar (a disaccharide composed of a molecule of glucose and fructose), are rapidly broken down by the body, resulting in a more rapid increase in blood glucose levels.

It is also important to recognise that some foods contain substances or compounds that can slow the absorption of carbohydrates. Dietary fibre, for example, reduces the rate at which carbohydrates are absorbed, and whole grains have a higher amount of dietary fibre than processed carbohydrates. Certain herbs or other foods, such as white beans, also contain compounds that slow the digestion of carbohydrates, which can aid in diabetes management. This suggests that some foods are more beneficial for individuals with diabetes than others.

Glycaemic Index (GI) and Glycaemic Load (GL)

The real question now is: how can we determine which foods are more suitable for people with diabetes and which are not? Learning about the nutritional profile of each food, including the content of various organic compounds, is a difficult, if not impossible, task.

To simplify things, researchers introduced the concepts of the glycaemic index (GI) and glycaemic load (GL).

When living with diabetes, it is important to consume foods that cause a slow increase in blood glucose, allowing the body sufficient time to utilise this glucose and thereby prevent insulin resistance.

The Glycaemic Index (GI)

This is a measure of how quickly any food causes a rise in blood glucose levels. Foods with a low glycaemic index are beneficial for preventing and managing diabetes (foods with a high glycaemic index (GI) should be avoided).

What are High and Low Glycaemic Indexes?

- **High-GI foods (GI 70 or above):** These foods are digested and absorbed quickly, resulting in a rapid increase in blood sugar levels.

- **Low-GI foods (GI 55 or below):** These foods are digested and absorbed more slowly, resulting in a gradual rise in blood sugar levels.

Examples of High- and Low-Glycaemic Index Foods.

High-GI Foods (GI ≥ 70)

Foods with a glycaemic index (GI) of 70 or higher raise blood sugar quickly. For example, **white bread** can cause a rapid increase in blood sugar; therefore, it is best to avoid it or consume it in small amounts. **Jasmine rice** is a variety of fragrant rice that digests quickly and can also lead to blood sugar spikes. **Cornflakes**, a type of processed cereal, noticeably impacts blood sugar levels. **Watermelon** is a natural fruit, but it has a high glycaemic index (GI); therefore, it is best to eat it alongside protein or fat to help balance its effects. **Baked potatoes** are high in starch and digest rapidly, so portion control is important. **Pretzels,** which are refined snacks, can also cause a swift rise in blood sugar levels.

Low-GI Foods (GI ≤ 55)

Foods with a low glycaemic index (GI) score of 55 or lower release glucose more slowly and steadily. **Lentils** are beneficial for maintaining stable blood sugar levels because of their high protein and fibre content. **Chickpeas** are also rich in protein and fibre, which helps sustain steady blood sugar levels. **Rolled oats** take a long time to digest, providing a lasting source of energy. **Apples** contain fibre and natural sugars; therefore, they have little impact on blood sugar. **Sweet potatoes** are nutrient-dense and increase glucose absorption more effectively than regular potatoes. Another low-GI item that helps keep blood sugar levels stable is **non-fat yoghurt**, which is high in protein.

There are many online databases and apps one can use to learn more about the glycaemic index of foods.

One such excellent online database is: *https://glycemicindex. com/gi-search/*

Please note that understanding the glycaemic index of foods alone is not enough and only part of the picture. Researchers soon realised that some foods with a high glycaemic index (GI), such as watermelon, are not necessarily bad for those living with diabetes, and some foods with a low glycaemic index (GI) are not necessarily good for them either. So, the GI of food alone cannot be the only factor to consider when choosing the appropriate foods for those living with diabetes.

Some foods may have fast-absorbing carbohydrates but contain very few carbohydrates, resulting in a very low glycaemic load (GL).

This means that for a complete picture, it is vital to consider both the glycaemic index (GI) and the glycaemic load (GL) of foods.

What is the Glycaemic Load?

The glycaemic load (GL) indicates the amount of sugar in any food and how long it takes to raise blood sugar levels.

Understanding how quickly any food raises blood sugar levels (glycaemic index, or GI) offers only partial information. However, considering both the glycaemic index (GI) and the glycaemic load (GL) gives a complete picture.

The Glycaemic Load (GL)

The glycaemic load (GL) considers both the glycaemic index (GI) and the carbohydrate content of food per serving.

What are High and Low Glycaemic Loads?

- **High-GL foods (GL 20 or above):** A typical serving of these foods causes a significant rise in blood sugar.
- **Low-GL foods (GL 10 or below):** A typical serving has little effect on blood sugar levels.

Examples of Foods with High and Low Glycaemic Loads

Foods with a high GL (GL ≥ 20 per serving):

- White rice (1 cup cooked) can quickly elevate blood sugar; therefore, it is best to limit your intake.
- A bagel (1 medium) is a dense, refined carbohydrate that can raise blood sugar levels.
- Raisins (¼ cup) are a rich source of natural sugar. To balance them out, consume them with protein or fat.
- A baked potato (1 medium) is starchy and easy to digest; add fibre or protein to it.
- Cornflakes (1 cup) are ultra-processed cereals that quickly raises blood sugar.
- A French baguette (slice) is a type of refined bread that can quickly raise blood sugar levels.

Foods with a low GL (GL ≤ 10 per serving:

- A medium-sized carrot is a whole, minimally processed food that provides a substantial amount of dietary fibre and has a low glycaemic load, resulting in a minimal increase in blood glucose levels following consumption.
- Kidney beans (½ cup cooked) are high in fibre and protein and release glucose steadily.

- Peanuts (1 oz) are low in carbohydrates, high in protein and healthy fats; helps maintain steady blood sugar levels. (Avoid if you have a peanut allergy).

- Grapefruit (1/2 medium) is a natural fruit with a low glycaemic index, making it suitable for maintaining stable blood sugar levels. (Avoid grapefruit if you are also taking cholesterol-lowering drugs).

- Cherries (1 cup) are a fruit that takes a long time to digest and does not raise blood sugar levels much.

- 1 cup of low-fat milk is high in protein and low in GL, which helps keep your energy levels constant.

The same database that provides information about glycaemic index (GI) also includes details on the glycaemic load (GL) of foods.

By considering both the glycaemic index (GI) and the glycaemic load (GL), individuals can choose a wider variety of foods, helping in the prevention and management of diabetes.

Search for glycaemic load of foods here: *https://glycemicindex. com/gi-search/*

CHAPTER 4
BUILDING A DIABETIC-FRIENDLY PLATE

At this stage, you have gained a comprehensive understanding of the nutritional science behind effective dietary practices for managing type 2 diabetes. This foundational knowledge allows you to critically evaluate carbohydrate quality and choose foods that support glycaemic control. Specifically, your awareness of the glycaemic index (GI) and glycaemic load (GL) provides you with a practical framework for structuring balanced meals and managing postprandial blood glucose levels.

The Plate Method

According to the American Diabetes Association (n.d.), the plate method is an easy, visual tool based on nutrition science and widely recommended by diabetes educators. Instead of measuring every gram or obsessively counting calories, this approach turns the dinner plate into a simple guide for creating balanced meals.

Imagine your plate is divided into two halves. One-half of the plate should be filled with non-starchy vegetables, such as broccoli, spinach, tomatoes, bell peppers, carrots, or salad greens. These foods are rich in fibre, vitamins, and minerals but low in carbohydrates. They help moderate blood sugar responses and support gut health.

The remaining half of the plate is divided equally between lean proteins and complex carbohydrates, also known as starchy foods.

Lean proteins may include fish, chicken breast, eggs, tofu, or legumes. These options promote satiety, which is the feeling of fullness and satisfaction after a meal, and help maintain muscle mass, both of which are vital for metabolic health.

For the last quarter, choose whole grains such as whole grain bread, barley, oats, and brown rice, or starchy vegetables like sweet potatoes or corn. These provide energy, but when properly combined with fibre and protein, they have a less significant impact on blood sugar levels.

Additionally, opt for water or zero-calorie drinks.

Breakdown of the Plate Method

- Vegetables (non-starchy) - 50%
- Complex carbohydrates – 25%
- Lean protein – 25%
- Water or zero-calorie drinks

To learn more about this eating pattern, visit the American Diabetes Association's website at: *https://diabetesfoodhub.org/blog/what-diabetes-plate*.

For more resources on healthy eating patterns for type 2 diabetes and related information, visit Diabetes UK: www.diabetes.org.uk/living-with-diabetes/eating.

These websites, known for their trustworthy and evidence-based information, offer free resources to help you eat healthier, including meal planning advice, tasty recipes, and other useful materials that can be downloaded.

Eating the right kind of food is beneficial, but it is also vital to eat the right amount, and this is where portion control becomes important.

Research shows that people often underestimate how much food they eat, especially when dining out or snacking straight from the packet. Additionally, studies have also confirmed that individuals tend to underestimate the calorie content of food, particularly in snacks or when eating out [7].

Mindful Eating

Mindful eating is a method of portion control that encourages you to be fully present during your meals, which has a profound impact on your overall health. By paying close attention to your hunger and fullness cues, savouring the flavours and textures of your meals, and avoiding distractions, you can cultivate a healthier relationship with food and gain a deeper appreciation for the nourishment it provides. Mindful eating can help you enjoy your food more, control your weight, and reduce overeating.

Simple habits, such as using smaller plates, serving food in the kitchen instead of at the table, or pausing halfway through a meal to check in with your appetite, can significantly reduce overeating. Other strategies include eating slowly, chewing food thoroughly, and taking smaller bites.

There are many ways to practice mindful eating. One effective method is to slow down and savour each bite. Eating too quickly gives the body less time to register fullness, making it easier to consume excess calories without realising. By taking the time to chew thoroughly and appreciate each bite, individuals not only enjoy their food more but may also experience improved digestion and greater meal satisfaction.

Studies suggest that individuals who practice mindful eating are more likely to maintain a healthy weight and better glycaemic control [8].

Finally, remember that you are what you eat, and you control what you put into your body. To make nutritional changes, start by adjusting your shopping habits. Prefer fresh produce, low-fat dairy, and lean proteins. Plan your meals for the week, make a list, and stick to it to avoid impulse purchases of ultra-processed foods. Reading nutrition labels is essential: look for products with fewer ingredients and avoid those where sugar or refined grains are listed first.

Meal Prepping

Meal prepping saves time and promotes balanced choices, even on busy days. Preparing ingredients beforehand, such as washing and chopping vegetables, cooking whole grains, or dividing snacks, makes it much easier to assemble healthy meals quickly. Batch-cooking staples like beans or chicken breasts offers flexibility throughout the week. Freezing leftovers in individual portions can help prevent food waste and maintain portion control, making it more convenient to eat.

When these strategies are incorporated into daily routines, healthy eating becomes more achievable and sustainable. Every small choice, from how you fill your plate to the way you shop and prepare meals, adds up to make a notable difference in your long-term health.

The Guiding Principles for a Diabetes-Friendly Plate

- Prioritise foods that are low-GI and low-GL, such as whole grains, legumes, and non-starchy vegetables.
- Balance macronutrients: allocate 50% of the plate to non-starchy vegetables, 25% to lean proteins, and 25% to complex carbohydrates.
- Mind portion sizes to minimise excess calories.
- Choose minimally processed foods to maximise nutrient density.
- Meal prep saves time.

CHAPTER 5
WHAT TO EAT AND WHAT TO AVOID

There are many good and not-so-good foods for people living with type 2 diabetes. Providing a complete list is undoubtedly beyond the scope of this book, and that is not its aim. We prefer to explain the underlying principles of choosing healthy foods. However, it is always helpful to provide a list to get started, giving some idea of what to eat and what to avoid.

Let's examine a healthy food list, including looking at the best options for blood sugar management, foods to avoid, and other key considerations.

Best Foods for Managing Blood Sugar

These foods contain nutrients such as fibre, protein, healthy fats, and antioxidants that slow glucose absorption and support stable blood sugar levels.

Some examples include:

Lentils and beans, such as chickpeas, black beans, and green lentils, are excellent options. They are high in fibre and protein, which help keep you fuller for longer and assist in lowering blood sugar levels after meals.

Citrus fruits and berries, such as oranges, strawberries, and blueberries, are also a wise choice. They are high in fibre and antioxidants and do not cause significant spikes in blood sugar.

Seeds and nuts, including almonds, pistachios, and chia seeds, provide healthy fats and fibre. They are filling and help sustain stable blood sugar levels.

Lean protein, such as Greek yoghurt, eggs, tuna, salmon, and chicken breast, slows the absorption of carbohydrates and helps insulin work more effectively.

Non-starchy vegetables, such as broccoli, leafy greens, and okra, are especially beneficial. They are low in carbohydrates but high in fibre and water, which helps slow down your body's response to glucose.

Whole grains, such as steel-cut oats, quinoa, and barley, are digested more slowly thanks to their high fibre content. That means that they help keep your energy levels and blood sugar steady.

Healthy fats, like those in avocados and olive oil, help slow digestion and regulate blood sugar levels when eaten with carbohydrates.

Foods to Reduce or Avoid and Smarter Alternatives

These foods tend to cause a spike in blood sugar. The alternatives offer similar satisfaction without the glucose spike.

Refined cereals, white rice, and white bread can cause blood sugar levels to spike rapidly.

Smarter alternatives include whole-grain bread, brown rice, or steel-cut oats, which help maintain steady blood sugar levels.

Sugary drinks and fruit juices should be avoided because your body absorbs the added sugar they contain very quickly.

Smarter alternatives include water, unsweetened tea, or sparkling water.

Sweetened dairy products, such as flavoured yoghurt, contain hidden sugars and should be avoided.

Smarter alternatives include plain Greek yoghurt topped with fresh berries, which offers a delicious and nutritious choice.

Fried snacks and pastries contain unhealthy fats and refined carbohydrates, which are harmful to your health.

Smarter alternatives include a crunchy and satisfying snack, such as roasted chickpeas or whole-grain crackers paired with hummus.

Full-fat dairy products, when consumed excessively, may pose problems due to their high saturated fat and calorie content.

Smarter alternatives include opting for low-fat options or controlling portion sizes, which is a more practical approach.

Ultra-processed foods labelled as **'diabetic-friendly'** can be misleading because they often contain high levels of sugar and unnecessary ingredients.

Smarter alternatives include whole foods, such as fruits, vegetables, lean meats, and legumes, which are the preferred choices.

Practical Food Swaps for Real-Life Meals

Here are simple changes that can make meals more diabetes-friendly without losing enjoyment.

- Making small, thoughtful changes can help keep your blood sugar levels stable. Instead of white rice, try quinoa or cauliflower rice, for instance. These options contain more fibre and nutrients, and significantly fewer processed carbohydrates.

- You do not have to give up pasta if you enjoy it. Just switch to whole-grain spaghetti or zucchini noodles. Both have a lower glycaemic index, more fibre, and help your body respond to glucose more slowly.

- Instead of sugary cereals, choose steel-cut oats or unsweetened muesli with berries, which contain less sugar, more fibre, and provide longer-lasting energy.

- Sweetened drinks can rapidly increase blood sugar levels. Instead, you can stay hydrated without adding sugar by drinking infused water or herbal iced tea.

- You can also choose whole-wheat or corn tortillas, paired with plenty of vegetables, as a healthier alternative to refined flour tortillas. These are higher in fibre and help prevent blood sugar levels from rising too quickly.

- If you usually buy fruit smoothies from the supermarket, consider switching to whole fruit with plain Greek yoghurt. This way, you get fibre with added protein and avoid the hidden sugars found in many ready-made smoothies.

These small changes help us make better food choices and maintain stable blood sugar levels in a way that is both realistic and sustainable.

PART

III

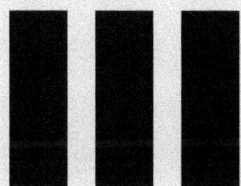

LIFESTYLE HABITS THAT SUPPORT BLOOD SUGAR BALANCE

CHAPTER 6
THE POWER OF PHYSICAL ACTIVITY

The most essential step in preventing and managing diabetes is making dietary changes. The second most vital step is regular exercise, which not only helps burn calories but also enhances overall well-being. Consider adding a short 10-minute walk to your routine to boost energy levels and lift your mood for the next hour. Emphasising such immediate benefits can make exercise seem like a reward rather than a chore.

However, it is important to recognise that exercise is not just about weight loss or managing diabetes; it offers numerous health benefits, including improved mood, stronger cardiovascular health, better blood circulation, and more, as well as lowering blood glucose levels and burning fat.

One reason metabolic disorders, once uncommon, have become so prevalent is that people move less nowadays. They lead sedentary lifestyles. The human body was designed to move and engage in physical activities every day. However, most jobs today do not require physical effort, making exercise even more crucial.

Furthermore, the skeletal muscles make up 40% of the body weight in a typical adult with normal weight[9]. Skeletal muscles are key consumers of glucose. Therefore, if individuals do not engage in sufficient physical activity during the day, it can lead to a notable decline in energy requirements.

The skeletal muscles utilise most of the carbohydrates we consume, playing a crucial role in regulating blood sugar levels. In people with diabetes, these muscles often become resistant to insulin, making it harder for them to absorb and store glucose as glycogen. Regular exercise helps reverse this process by improving insulin sensitivity and enhancing the muscle's ability to both store and burn glucose.

It is worth noting that muscle mass also plays a role, making resistance training very important. If you have more muscle mass, you can burn more calories in less time. Obese people have a lot of fat tissue and less muscle mass, which explains why they find it difficult to lose weight.

An effective exercise plan should include a combination of resistance and aerobic training.

Best Types of Exercise for Type 2 Diabetes

Regular physical activity delivers powerful benefits for individuals with type 2 diabetes:

- **Aerobic exercise** (e.g., brisk walking, swimming, cycling, dancing) improves blood glucose levels, enhances insulin sensitivity, supports cardiovascular health, and complements weight management goals.
- **Resistance training** (e.g., weightlifting, resistance bands, bodyweight exercises) helps build and preserve muscle mass, increasing glucose uptake and insulin sensitivity.
- **High-intensity interval training** (HIIT), which involves short bursts of high-intensity exercise followed by recovery periods,

can effectively and efficiently improve glucose metabolism. However, it may not be suitable for everyone and should be undertaken with the supervision of a healthcare professional.

- **Light, gentle movement** (e.g., yoga, tai chi, post-meal walks) enhances balance and flexibility and reduces postprandial glucose spikes without stressing the body.

Creating a Sustainable Fitness Routine

Remember that establishing a lasting exercise habit relies on personalisation, variety, timing, and practicality. To bridge the gap between intention and action, consider adding simple 'if-then' plans to your routine. For example, using phrases like 'If I finish dinner, then I will walk for 10 minutes' can turn advice into automatic habit triggers. This method can make these actions more instinctive, supporting consistency and motivation.

- **Combine cardio and strength training:** Aim for at least 150 minutes of moderate aerobic activity per week, plus 2–3 sessions of strength training. This blend yields stronger glucose control and greater health benefits.

- **Timing matters—post-meal activity:** Exercising after meals, especially in the evening, can help reduce blood sugar spikes and may even improve morning fasting glucose levels.

- **Short, frequent sessions work:** Splitting activity into 10–15-minute post-meal sessions can be as practical, or even superior, to longer, less frequent workouts.

- **Mix it up:** Switching between aerobic, resistance, and flexibility exercises keeps routines engaging, targets various aspects of fitness, and adapts to changing daily schedules.

- **Start small and build:** Begin with simple, enjoyable movements such as walking or gentle stretching, gradually increasing the frequency, duration, and intensity. Consistency is more important than intensity, especially in the early stages of training.

- **Include everyday movements:** Incorporate routine activities such as taking the stairs, walking short errands on foot, or engaging in light gardening. These choices help reduce sedentary behaviour and encourage healthy habits.

- **Consult with professionals:** Tailor your plan to your abilities, risk factors, and preferences by consulting your healthcare or fitness specialists, especially if you are managing complications such as neuropathy or heart conditions.

Brief Summary

Best exercises: Incorporate a well-rounded mix of aerobic, strength, HIIT, and gentle movement exercises.

- **Sustainability tips**: Align your routine with your personal preferences. Break sessions into manageable pieces, vary your activities, and emphasise consistency.

- **Smart timing:** Choose post-meal activities whenever possible for better blood sugar control.

Start slowly, listen to your body, and develop a routine that fits your lifestyle. Before starting any new exercise programme, it is essential to consult a healthcare professional to ensure safety and maximise benefits.

CHAPTER 7
STRESS AND SLEEP

Chronic stress and diabetes

Stress, particularly chronic stress, is a recognised cause of insulin resistance. It is vital to understand that acute and chronic stress differ significantly.

Acute stress mainly acts as a defence mechanism, activating the 'fight or flight' response. Adrenaline is the primary hormone involved in this response, which usually lasts for a few minutes.

However, the chronic stress response is entirely different. Experts compare it to constantly pressing the alarm button. This prolonged stress can cause serious harm to someone's health, yet it may not show noticeable symptoms in its early stages and often remains largely unnoticed.

Chronic stress, such as work-related stress, ongoing financial difficulties, relationship issues, or other factors, raises cortisol levels.

Cortisol is a gluco-corticosteroid hormone that is known to suppress immunity, weaken bones, increase blood glucose levels (by increasing glucagon production), contribute to insulin resistance, and damage cardiovascular health. All these harmful effects occur slowly over months and years, and many people fail to realise that their health issues are due to chronic stress [10].

This, therefore, means that stress management should be a vital aspect of preventing and controlling diabetes; fortunately, several well-researched techniques can help soothe both the mind and body.

Deep Controlled Breathing

One effective way to manage stress is through deep, controlled breathing. Although it seems simple, taking slow, deep breaths signals your nervous system to relax. Try inhaling slowly for four seconds, holding your breath for four seconds, then exhaling for six to eight seconds. Doing this for a few minutes can considerably decrease tension. Avoid if you have a heart condition, breathing pattern disorders, or after specific injuries or surgeries. Suppose you experience dizziness, chest pain, shortness of breath, or a panic sensation while deep breathing, stop immediately and seek medical attention.

Progressive Muscle Relaxation

Another practical approach is progressive muscle relaxation. This involves tensing and then relaxing different muscle groups in sequence, from your toes up to your shoulders. As you focus on releasing tension, your body naturally shifts away from 'fight or flight' mode to a calm, relaxed mode.

Mindfulness Meditation

People also widely recommend mindfulness meditation. The idea is to pay attention to the present moment, your breath, sensations, or even the sounds around you, without judgment. Research shows that just ten minutes a day can help lower anxiety and even improve blood sugar control.

Physical Activity

Physical activity, like a brisk walk, dancing, or gardening, naturally helps to relieve stress. Movement promotes the release of feel-good endorphins and clears the mind. Even a quick stretch or gentle yoga can boost your mood.

Social Support

Do not underestimate social support either. Spending time with friends, talking with a loved one, or joining a support group can provide perspective and remind you that you are not alone.

Laughter, Hobbies, Time in Nature

Ultimately, laughter, hobbies, and spending time in nature all contribute to breaking the cycle of stress.

The key is to find a few techniques that work for you and incorporate them into your daily routine.

The Importance of Sleep and Tips for Sleep Hygiene

Sleep is not just a time to rest; it is when the body resets vital functions, including hormone balance and blood sugar regulation. Poor sleep has also been linked to increased insulin resistance and higher blood glucose levels, even in people without diabetes.

Adults typically require seven to nine hours of high-quality sleep each night. However, it is not just about how much sleep you get; quality is important too. Creating a comfortable sleep environment, sticking to a regular sleep routine, and establishing a calming bedtime ritual can significantly improve sleep quality.

Good sleep hygiene involves establishing habits and routines that promote quality sleep. First, try to go to bed and wake up at the same time each day, even on weekends. This keeps your body clock in sync.

Create a soothing wind-down routine before bed: dim the lights, avoid screens for at least 30 minutes to an hour before bedtime, and engage in a relaxing activity such as reading or listening to music. Keep your bedroom calm, dark, and quiet. Blackout curtains, a fan, or white noise can help.

Limit caffeine consumption in the afternoon and avoid large meals or heavy snacks just before bedtime. Alcohol might initially make you sleepy, but it disrupts sleep quality as the night unfolds.

If you wake during the night, try not to watch the clock or reach for your phone. Instead, focus on your breathing or try a short relaxation technique until you feel sleepy again.

If you continue to experience persistent trouble sleeping, please consult your healthcare professional. Addressing sleep issues can significantly improve your energy, mood, and diabetes management.

Small improvements in stress management and sleep routines add up, helping you feel and perform at your best each day.

CHAPTER 8
WEIGHT MANAGEMENT WITHOUT FAD DIETING

I n many European and other high-income countries, more than half the population is overweight. Consequently, obesity has become the primary cause of type 2 diabetes and several other non-communicable diseases. Effectively managing weight can therefore help prevent many cases of diabetes.

In many countries today, obesity is increasingly recognised as a disease rather than just a risk factor for other diseases [11].

Weight management should be a key part of diabetes care. However, it does not mean dieting and risking malnutrition. We advise against fad diets, as most are unsustainable and may even lead to other health problems.

There are many healthier ways to lose weight, including reducing total calorie intake while ensuring that the diet contains all necessary nutrients. Dietary measures, such as controlling portion sizes and understanding what makes up a healthy plate, as previously discussed, can aid in weight management and diabetes control.

Nutritional measures, when combined with exercise and stress management, can help individuals lose weight in many cases.

Why Weight Loss Can Improve Blood Sugar Control

It is essential to recognise that for people with type 2 diabetes or at risk of developing it, even modest weight loss can significantly improve blood sugar control. When the body accumulates excess fat, particularly around the abdomen, it becomes more difficult for insulin to transport glucose from the blood into the cells, where it can be utilised for energy. Additionally, belly fat secretes adipokines, which are known to cause inflammation and worsen diabetes [12]

You do not have to lose a large amount of body weight to enjoy health benefits, lower the risk of diabetes, or improve blood glucose levels. In fact, studies show that losing as little as five to ten per cent of your initial weight can improve insulin resistance and enable your body's insulin to work more effectively [13]. This suggests that even small, manageable changes can make a significant difference, empowering you to take control of your health.

Furthermore, highlighting changes in body composition, such as a reduction in waist circumference or an increase in muscle mass, can give a more comprehensive view of progress. These measurements can help you evaluate success more accurately than just focusing on weight loss, keeping you motivated even when the scales do not reflect your efforts (Ludwig, 2016).

Losing weight can enhance insulin sensitivity. Insulin sensitivity refers to how effectively your cells can absorb glucose from the blood. When you are overweight, your cells may become resistant to insulin, resulting in higher blood sugar levels. However, by losing some weight, your cells can absorb glucose more efficiently, which can lead to lower blood sugar levels. Sometimes, initial weight loss can delay or prevent the need for diabetes medication. For those with prediabetes, weight loss is one of the most effective ways to reduce the risk of developing full-blown diabetes.

Healthy Strategies for Weight Loss and Maintenance

The most effective weight loss strategies are gradual, realistic, and rooted in habits you can sustain long-term. Crash diets or extreme calorie restrictions may produce quick results, but they rarely last and can even be harmful.

Healthy Eating

Begin with simple adjustments: concentrate on eating regular, balanced meals using the plate method. This approach has already been discussed in 'Chapter 4'. This balanced technique ensures you obtain a variety of nutrients and helps regulate portion sizes. Choose foods high in fibre, such as beans, whole grains, and vegetables, as these help keep you full and stabilise your blood sugar. Be aware of liquid calories from sugary drinks, which can accumulate rapidly.

Tracking your food intake, setting small, achievable goals, and celebrating progress along the way can help keep you motivated.

Physical Activity

Physical activity is vital, not only for burning calories but also for maintaining muscle mass and increasing metabolism. Aim for at least 150 minutes of moderate-intensity exercise each week and include strength training at least twice a week to help your body preserve muscle while reducing fat.

Sleep and Stress Management

It is also crucial to get enough sleep and manage stress, as both can influence hunger hormones and cravings.

Maintenance

Once you reach your goal, concentrate on maintaining rather than continuing to lose weight. Keep up with regular physical activity, keep portion sizes reasonable, and regularly review your eating habits to stay on track.

Remember, these changes are not just for now, but for your long-term health and well-being. Every healthy choice you make supports better blood sugar levels and a brighter future.

Managing Plateaus

Almost everyone encounters a plateau at some stage, a period when weight loss stalls, even though you are still doing the right things. This can be frustrating, but it is a normal part of the process. Remember, you are not alone in this journey, and these plateaus are a common part of it. Keep going, and you will see progress once again.

Plateaus occur because, as you lose weight, your body requires fewer calories to sustain its new size, and metabolism may slow down slightly.

To overcome a plateau, it helps to assess your habits and make the necessary adjustments. Are your portions gradually increasing? Has your activity level decreased? Sometimes, minor changes like altering your exercise routine, adding a few extra minutes of movement, or paying closer attention to portion sizes can restart your progress.

It is also essential to be patient. Plateaus can last from a few weeks to several months. Focus on the positive health improvements you have achieved, not just the number on the scale. Remember, maintaining weight loss is an accomplishment, and every healthy choice supports better blood sugar control and long-term well-being.

Stay consistent, stay kind to yourself, and trust the process. Progress is not always linear, but every step matters.

CHAPTER 9
LIMITING ALCOHOL AND SMOKING CESSATION

M anaging or preventing type 2 diabetes involves more than just watching what you eat, being more physically active, and monitoring your blood sugar levels. Two lifestyle choices often go unnoticed: alcohol consumption and smoking. Both can significantly influence blood sugar control and long-term health, whether you aim to prevent diabetes or manage it effectively.

The Role of Alcohol in Diabetes

Alcohol does not directly cause diabetes, but regular or excessive drinking can increase your risk. Heavy drinking may reduce your body's sensitivity to insulin, shifting the balance towards type 2 diabetes. High alcohol consumption can also lead to chronic pancreatitis, which might itself cause diabetes, and the calories from drinks, often overlooked, can contribute to weight gain, a well-known risk factor [14].

For those already living with diabetes, alcohol brings its own set of challenges. Alcohol can interfere with the liver's ability to regulate blood sugar, increasing the risk of hypoglycaemia, especially for people taking insulin or certain blood sugar-lowering medications.

Moderation is crucial. The American Diabetes Association (ADA) emphasises that alcohol consumption decisions should be personalised [15]. Factors such as your medications, blood sugar control, weight, and overall health are important considerations (Alcohol and Diabetes, n.d.). Discuss your concerns with your healthcare professional to evaluate the safety of your treatment. However, the World Health Organisation (WHO) released a statement published in The Lancet Public Health on 4 January 2023, stating that there is no safe level of alcohol consumption that benefits our health (No level of alcohol consumption is safe for our health, 2023).

Smoking and Diabetes Risk

Smoking is arguably one of the most overlooked risk factors for diabetes.

Research indicates that active smokers have a 30–40% higher likelihood of developing type 2 diabetes compared to non-smokers. The World Health Organisation (WHO) considers smoking a modifiable risk factor in diabetes prevention [16]. (Quitting smoking reduces your risk of developing type 2 diabetes by 30–40%, 2023).

For people already living with diabetes, quitting smoking not only reduces future risk but also brings immediate benefits. UK government data show that within just one year of quitting, the risk of hospitalisation due to a heart attack drops by 67%. Within five years, cardiovascular mortality falls by up to 45%, bringing risk closer to that of non-smokers [17].

Quitting smoking also lowers the risk of serious diabetes-related complications, such as kidney disease and poor vascular health, regardless of any accompanying weight gain.

Putting It All Together

Excessive alcohol consumption and tobacco smoking significantly increase diabetes risk. They also increase the risk of diabetes-related complications.

The good news? Both quitting smoking and reducing alcohol intake for those who do not want to stop altogether are powerful, actionable steps. They make a tangible difference even without other changes.

Practical Step Forward

1. Set realistic limits with alcohol. It is best to exercise caution. The World Health Organisation (WHO) emphasises that no level of alcohol consumption is truly safe for health. However, many national health authorities provide unit-based guidelines to help minimise harm for those who choose to continue drinking. If you consume alcohol, seek help to stop or aim to stay within your government's recommended weekly limits, spread intake over several days, and include alcohol-free intervals. Since alcohol can affect blood sugar and interact with diabetes medications, it is wise to discuss your individual circumstances with your healthcare professional.

2. Create safety nets. Carry hypo treats if at risk, wear a medical ID, and inform close friends or family members about what to do if your blood sugar levels drop.

3. Quit smoking and seek help. Even occasional tobacco smoking is harmful. If you find it challenging to quit smoking, seek help.

4. Rely on your healthcare team. Be open about challenges, whether it is reducing or stopping alcohol or quitting smoking. Together, you can create a step-by-step plan that works for you.

By tackling alcohol and smoking thoughtfully, you are not just reducing the risk of developing type 2 diabetes; you are giving your body a better chance to manage it effectively. One small change, one day at a time, can shift the balance toward lasting health.

PART

IV

LIVING WELL WITH DIABETES

CHAPTER 10
PARTNERING WITH YOUR HEALTHCARE TEAM

L ifestyle interventions form a key part of the overall strategy to prevent and manage diabetes. Even if you have severe diabetes, these simple lifestyle changes can make a meaningful difference. They not only help prevent the progression of diabetes but also reduce the risk of complications. People living with diabetes should practise these interventions, continue taking their medications, and work closely with their healthcare team.

Making Informed Choices for Type 2 Diabetes Management

Living well with type 2 diabetes is more about consistently making informed choices than following strict rules. Each day presents opportunities to improve your health, whether deciding what to have for breakfast, how to move your body, or how to manage stress. At the centre of this is knowledge: understanding your body, your condition, and the many tools available to help you manage it. This knowledge empowers you, giving you the confidence to make the best decisions for your health.

An informed choice starts with reliable information. For instance, knowing how different foods affect your blood sugar can help you build balanced meals that not only satisfy your taste buds but also support glucose control. This includes reading nutrition labels, being aware of carbohydrate content, and appreciating the effects of fibre, fat, and protein on digestion. It means recognising that some foods, even those marketed as 'healthy' or 'natural,' may contain hidden sugars or highly refined grains that can spike your blood sugar.

Beyond food, informed choices also include movement, stress management, and sleep. You don't need to run marathons or overhaul your entire lifestyle overnight. Instead, focus on small, realistic adjustments, such as adding a ten-minute walk after dinner, practising mindfulness, or establishing a regular sleep routine. Consistency in these choices has a greater impact than perfection.

Nevertheless, even with good intentions and consistent effort, managing blood sugar is not always simple. Genetics, age, hormonal shifts, and other health conditions can all affect how your body responds. For some, lifestyle changes alone might not be enough to keep blood glucose levels within a healthy range.

Considering Medications When Needed

Needing medication for type 2 diabetes is not a failure; it is simply an acknowledgement that diabetes is a complex, progressive condition. Over time, the body may produce less insulin or use it less effectively, even if you are eating well and staying active. In these cases, oral medications or injectable therapies can provide essential support.

The decision to start medication varies based on individual factors. Your healthcare professional will consider your blood sugar patterns, personal health history, lifestyle, and preferences to determine the most appropriate course of action.

For many individuals, metformin is the first medication recommended. It works by reducing the amount of sugar produced by the liver and increasing the body's sensitivity to insulin. Your healthcare team may adjust or change your medications based on your individual needs, such as lowering cardiovascular risk, supporting weight management, or reducing side effects. They may also recommend newer options, such as GLP-1 receptor agonists (e.g., semaglutide) or SGLT2 inhibitors (e.g., empagliflozin), earlier in treatment, especially if you have a higher cardiovascular or kidney risk.

Many people worry about needing medication and associate it with worsening health. Starting medication when necessary is a sensible approach. Early and effective blood sugar control can help prevent complications such as nerve damage, kidney disease, and vision loss. Medications are not 'either/or' tools; they work best when viewed as part of a comprehensive approach, alongside nutrition, exercise, and stress management.

Combining Medication and Lifestyle for Optimal Control

The most effective strategies for managing type 2 diabetes combine medication and lifestyle, rather than relying on one at the expense of the other. Think of it as teamwork: medication addresses the underlying physiology, helping your body produce, release, or use insulin more effectively, while lifestyle habits influence how much glucose enters your bloodstream and how well your body can manage it.

For example, medications like SGLT2 inhibitors help remove excess glucose through the urine, while healthy eating ensures you are not overwhelming your system with large sugar loads. Regular physical activity improves insulin sensitivity, enabling both your body and medications to function more effectively. Even stress reduction and adequate sleep can reduce insulin resistance and support the effectiveness of your medication.

Regular monitoring is essential to maintaining the right balance. Please keep a record of your blood glucose levels, observe how they respond to meals, activity, and medication, and share these patterns with your healthcare team. Being proactive is vital for managing your diabetes effectively. Over time, adjustments may be needed. The aim is not just to achieve a specific number, but to support your overall well-being and quality of life.

It is crucial to communicate openly with your healthcare professional about how you are feeling, any side effects, or concerns regarding your treatment plan. Ask questions, share successes and setbacks, and collaborate to adjust your approach as life evolves.

Informed choices, openness to medication when necessary, and a commitment to holistic self-care enable you to manage type 2 diabetes confidently. While an individual's journey is unique, the right knowledge, coupled with a flexible and supportive approach, makes achieving optimal blood sugar control both realistic and sustainable.

CHAPTER 11
TRACKING YOUR PROGRESS

Diabetes is not just about high blood glucose levels. It causes numerous health problems. Most people with diabetes have high bad cholesterol, high blood pressure, an increased risk of heart disease, neuropathy, and more. Diabetes is the leading cause of chronic kidney disease, poorly healing ulcers, and various other problems. Therefore, it is vital to closely monitor various health parameters, which can help you take timely actions to prevent the development and worsening of diabetes-related complications.

The actual value of ongoing monitoring is not just in the numbers themselves but in what those numbers reveal about your health and your ability to prevent complications before they arise. In type 2 diabetes, this involves closely tracking blood sugar levels but also looking beyond glucose to other health indicators that can change silently over time.

Blood glucose self-monitoring, using a glucometer or a continuous glucose monitor (CGM), provides real-time feedback on how meals, physical activity, illness, and stress influence your body. This information is vital for making daily decisions about food, exercise, and medication, as well as recognising both high and low blood sugar levels before they cause harm. For those on insulin or medications that can cause hypoglycaemia, regular blood sugar checks are essential for safety. Even people not using these medications can benefit from occasional testing, as it helps to identify patterns and guide long-term choices.

Haemoglobin A1C, typically measured in a laboratory, offers a broader overview. Unlike individual glucose readings, A1C reflects the average blood sugar control over the past two to three months. This test helps you and your healthcare professional evaluate whether your overall management plan is practical, not just for today but over time. A1C is also an important predictor of the risk of complications: the closer your reading is to the recommended target, the lower your risk of nerve damage, eye disease, and kidney issues.

Monitoring weight is another essential aspect. While the scale does not tell the whole story, unintentional weight gain or loss can indicate underlying issues. For many, modest weight loss can improve insulin sensitivity, lower blood glucose levels, and reduce the risk of cardiovascular disease. Tracking weight also helps evaluate the effects of dietary and physical activity changes and can alert the team if medication adjustments are necessary.

Blood pressure is closely linked to diabetes outcomes. Hypertension often coexists with diabetes and is a significant risk factor for heart attack, stroke, kidney damage, and eye disease. Regular blood pressure monitoring, both at home and in clinics, enables timely treatment and helps reduce the risk of serious health events. Studies have shown that effective blood pressure control and glucose management can significantly reduce the occurrence of microvascular and macrovascular complications.

Cholesterol and other blood lipids are monitored through blood tests, which are usually performed annually or more frequently if the results are abnormal. Elevated LDL cholesterol and triglycerides, along with low HDL, increase the risk of heart disease, a leading cause of death in people with diabetes. Tracking these markers enables early intervention through lifestyle changes or medications, such as statins, which help safeguard blood vessels and heart health.

Kidney health requires careful attention, as diabetes is the primary cause of chronic kidney disease globally. Consistently high blood sugar over time can damage the delicate filtration units in the kidneys. Blood tests for creatinine, used to estimate glomerular filtration rate (eGFR), and urine tests for albumin can detect early signs of stress on the kidney well before symptoms develop. Early detection is vital in slowing disease progression, making regular monitoring essential even when no symptoms are present.

Eye health should never be overlooked. Persistently elevated blood glucose can damage the retina, sometimes leading to vision loss. An eye specialist can identify retinopathy early through annual dilated retinal examinations, often before patients notice any changes in their vision. Timely intervention, whether through improved glucose control or ophthalmologic treatments, can prevent progression and preserve sight.

Nerve and foot health monitoring completes comprehensive care. High glucose levels over time can damage nerves and reduce circulation, particularly in the feet. This increases the risk of unnoticed injuries, infections, and even amputations. Daily self-examinations and annual professional foot assessments help identify any issues early, allowing for prompt treatment and ongoing education in foot care.

Each of these tests and assessments plays a unique, vital role in managing diabetes. Together, they create a safety net, providing both immediate feedback and long-term insight. They enable early detection of issues, informed decision-making, and the opportunity to personalise treatment as your diabetes and life evolve. Regular, thoughtful monitoring is not just about gathering data; it is an active, empowering process that supports your health and independence for many years to come.

Remember, it is about making informed choices, seeking help when needed, and working closely with your healthcare team. They are there to support and guide you. You are not alone on this journey.

Settings for Recommended Health Monitoring

Blood glucose is measured using a glucometer or a continuous glucose monitor at home or in a clinic. Self-monitoring is often recommended daily or as advised by your healthcare team, depending on what medication you are taking, to detect hypoglycaemia and hyperglycaemia, recognise patterns, and guide adjustments to diet, activity, and medication.

Haemoglobin A1C is assessed through a laboratory blood test every 3–6 months. This provides an average reading of glucose control over the previous 2–3 months and is a key indicator of long-term management.

Weight should be recorded using a scale at home or in a clinic. Patients may monitor their weight weekly or monthly at home. Clinicians usually measure it annually during the diabetes review, or more frequently if needed. Tracking weight helps identify trends and assess the effects of lifestyle interventions or medication.

Blood pressure is measured (manually or automatically) at home, in a clinic, or in a pharmacy. It should be checked at every clinic visit and at home if necessary. Regular monitoring allows for early detection and management of hypertension, thereby lowering the risk of cardiovascular and kidney disease.

Lipid profiles, including LDL, HDL, total cholesterol, and triglycerides, should be performed on an annual basis or more frequently if results are abnormal. Monitoring lipids helps assess cardiovascular risk and guides treatment options, such as statin therapy.

Kidney function is checked annually with a blood test for creatinine, urea, electrolytes (like sodium and potassium), glomerular filtration rate (eGFR), and protein (albumin) in urine, or more often if chronic kidney disease is present. Early detection of any abnormalities allows for timely intervention to slow their progression.

Eye health is assessed by an eye specialist with a yearly dilated retinal exam. This enables early detection and treatment of diabetic retinopathy, thereby reducing the risk of vision loss.

Foot and nerve health requires daily self-examination and an annual clinical check-up of the feet. This helps in early detection of neuropathy, poor circulation, or skin breakdown, and lowers the risk of ulceration, infection, and amputation.

Liver function is typically assessed annually through a blood test or monitored more frequently if abnormalities are detected. It helps to detect or screen for non-alcoholic fatty liver disease and medication side effects, as well as to evaluate the overall health of the liver. Early detection of potential issues enables timely intervention and management.

Dental health should be evaluated every six months by the dentist for early detection of gum disease, which is more common in people with diabetes and can impact glucose control.

Vaccinations such as the flu, pneumonia, and hepatitis B vaccines, as recommended, can be administered by your healthcare team in the clinic or at a pharmacy to help prevent infections that may be more severe in people with diabetes.

Note: The frequency of these tests or health checks may increase if results are abnormal or as directed by your healthcare professional or diabetes team.

Tools for Everyday Monitoring

Modern diabetes management provides many valuable tools:

Glucometer: compact, accurate, and simple to use. Including test strips and lancets, it enables regular home testing of capillary blood glucose.

Continuous Glucose Monitors (CGMs): Small sensors worn on the skin provide real-time glucose trends, reducing the need for finger-prick tests.

Blood pressure monitors: Affordable, home-use cuffs (both automatic and manual) are widely available, providing reliable readings.

Digital Food Journals & Apps: Smartphone apps help track food consumption, carbohydrate counts, exercise, weight, and even medication reminders. Logging meals can uncover patterns and triggers.

Traditional Journals: A straightforward notebook for recording blood glucose levels, meals, symptoms, or physical activity remains an effective, low-tech solution.

Wearable Fitness Trackers: Many devices now connect with apps to monitor steps, sleep, heart rate, and even glucose levels (if compatible with a Continuous Glucose Monitor, or CGM).

Adjusting Your Treatment Plan Over Time

Long-term management of type 2 diabetes requires regular reassessment and adjustment of the treatment plan as metabolic needs and individual circumstances change. Consider the case of Mrs Smith, a 57-year-old who initially maintained glycaemic control through dietary changes and regular exercise. Over several years, however, she noticed a gradual increase in her blood glucose levels and reported more fatigue despite sticking to her established routine. After consulting her healthcare team, they reviewed her self-monitoring records, diet, and activity patterns. Her clinician identified that age-related changes and a recent decrease in physical activity, resulting from a knee injury, contributed to the rising glucose levels. In response, her healthcare team collaborated to modify her meal plan, recommend low-impact aerobic exercises, and introduce a low-dose glucagon-like peptide-1 (GLP-1) receptor agonist to enhance blood glucose control.

This example highlights the importance of ongoing monitoring and personalised adjustments based on changing health status, comorbidities, and lifestyle modifications. Treatment plans may need to be adjusted in response to fluctuations in blood glucose levels, weight changes, the development of diabetes-related complications, or changes in life circumstances, such as physical limitations, psychological stress, or the initiation of new medications. Collaborative decision-making with healthcare professionals allows for timely and evidence-based modifications to therapeutic strategies, maximising both effectiveness and safety while supporting patient autonomy and quality of life.

Type 2 diabetes is not a fixed condition; it evolves as you do. Stress, ageing, changes in physical activity, new medications, and even life events can affect blood sugar patterns and other health metrics. That is why continuous monitoring is essential: it offers the information you need to adapt your plan in collaboration with your healthcare team.

Sometimes, that means adjusting meal plans or exercise routines. At other times, medications may need to be added, stopped, or adjusted. For example, if your A1C exceeds the target, your healthcare team may suggest a medication with additional cardiovascular or kidney benefits, depending on your individual circumstances. Your healthcare team may also consider new therapies or lifestyle changes if your cholesterol or blood pressure levels increase.

Regular check-ins, both at home and in the clinic, allow you to celebrate successes and identify issues early, well before they cause complications. Remember, even small changes can make a big difference. The key is to stay engaged, remain curious about your health data, and maintain open lines of communication with your healthcare team.

CHAPTER 12
STAYING MOTIVATED

This book presents extensive evidence from clinical studies demonstrating that lifestyle interventions are highly effective in preventing type 2 diabetes and promoting remission. However, applying these recommendations in daily life remains challenging for many individuals. The main challenges in staying motivated include difficulties with planning and sticking to the recommended plan.

Maintaining motivation over extended periods is especially challenging, as initial enthusiasm for lifestyle change can wane.

To maintain engagement, individuals are encouraged to monitor specific habits, such as the number of consecutive days without consuming sugary drinks, and to visualise their progress to boost motivation. Recognising and celebrating small achievements offers positive reinforcement and can enhance the consistency needed for lasting behavioural change.

Consider setting tangible, small milestones to stay highly motivated. For example, imagine a '7-day streak badge' system, where you reward yourself after consistently following your plan for a week.

To focus and sustain motivation, identify one keystone habit that offers multiple benefits. This could include maintaining a regular sleep routine, setting a daily step count goal, or practising consistent meal prep.

Track this keystone habit on a simple calendar, marking daily successes to reinforce your progress visually.

Recognising small wins can boost self-efficacy and help maintain your long-term commitment to lifestyle changes. Celebrating these mini milestones can create a strong foundation for reaching your ultimate health goals.

As we move on, we will focus on the practical aspects of getting started with lifestyle interventions and provide tips for staying motivated. When people practice lifestyle interventions consistently over time, they can experience significant health benefits.

Remember, type 2 diabetes often develops over many years of neglect and unhealthy dietary and lifestyle habits. Reversing the effects of these choices can take months or even years, but the effort is undoubtedly worthwhile. These changes not only help prevent or manage diabetes, but they can also add many healthy years to your life.

Setting SMART Goals

The SMART framework—Specific, Measurable, Achievable, Relevant, and Time-bound — is more than just a buzzword. It provides a simple structure for translating vague hopes into actionable steps.

Instead of saying, 'I want to exercise more,' a SMART goal would look like this: 'I will walk briskly for 20 minutes after dinner, five days a week, for the next month.' The goal is specific (walking briskly after dinner), measurable (20 minutes, five days a week), achievable (realistic for most), relevant (supports blood sugar control), and time-bound (for the next month). Consider treating each SMART goal as a 30-day trial, allowing yourself to adjust and learn as you go. This approach transforms the goal into an experiment rather than a pass-fail test, nurturing persistence through inevitable revisions.

Dealing with Setbacks

Even with the best goals and intentions, setbacks are inevitable. Life is unpredictable: illnesses, work demands, family issues, or even just low motivation can interrupt routines. The key is not to view setbacks as failures, but as part of the process. Everyone slips up now and then. What matters most is how you respond.

Instead of criticising yourself, practice self-compassion. Pause and reflect on what happened. Were your expectations too high, or did something unexpected throw you off course? Use setbacks as learning opportunities. Perhaps you realise that aiming to exercise every day is unrealistic, but three or four days a week is a more achievable goal. Alternatively, you may find that late-night snacking is most challenging when you are stressed, indicating a need for alternative coping strategies.

To stay prepared for future challenges, consider using a quick 'if-then' plan. For example, 'If the dessert menu is presented in a restaurant, then I will order green tea.' Practising these mental scripts in advance can boost your self-confidence and help you manage real-life temptations more effectively.

If you stray from your course, do not wait until the following Monday or the next month to start again; reset as soon as possible. Even a single healthy decision after a setback helps you stay on the right track. Remember, progress in health is seldom linear; it's normal for motivation to fluctuate. The key is to recommit regularly and not let one tough week turn into a lost month.

Building a Support System

No one succeeds alone. Building a strong support system is essential for making lasting changes. Support can take many forms, such as family members who walk with you, friends who share healthy recipes, online communities, or diabetes education groups. Even brief words of encouragement can make a difference on a difficult day.

Share your goals with those around you. This not only helps build accountability but also creates opportunities for practical support. Ask a friend to join you on morning walks or tell your partner that you would like to keep healthy snacks available. Healthcare professionals also form part of your support network. Diabetes educators, nutritionists, and doctors can offer guidance, answer questions, and adapt your plan as needed.

Social support also provides emotional resilience. When setbacks happen, loved ones can offer perspective and remind you of your successes. Sharing your experiences, both struggles and achievements, can reduce stress and reinforce motivation.

In summary, genuine progress comes from setting clear, achievable goals, learning from setbacks, and surrounding yourself with supportive people. These strategies lay a foundation not only for managing diabetes but also for thriving with it, day by day.

CHAPTER 13
SPECIAL CONSIDERATIONS

Diabetes rarely occurs alone. Many people with type 2 diabetes also need to manage other chronic conditions, such as high blood pressure, high cholesterol, cardiovascular disease, or polycystic ovary syndrome (PCOS). Most of these conditions are caused or worsened by diabetes.

It is essential to recognise that PCOS primarily involves insulin resistance, leading to hormonal imbalances. Similarly, poorly managed diabetes causes artery stiffening, resulting in high blood pressure and an increased risk of heart attack and stroke. Diabetes also elevates bad cholesterol levels, damages various organs and the nervous system, among many other issues. Therefore, managing multiple health conditions is crucial when living with diabetes.

However, each additional condition introduces its own challenges and risks, but understanding how they interact and addressing them together can greatly improve both daily well-being and long-term outcomes.

Managing Diabetes with Other Conditions

The most common companion to type 2 diabetes is **hypertension, or high blood pressure.** According to extensive studies, over two-thirds of adults with diabetes also have high blood pressure. The connection is not coincidental; both share common risk factors, including excess weight, physical inactivity, and insulin resistance.

Over time, elevated blood sugar and blood pressure together place extra strain on the heart, kidneys, eyes, and blood vessels, significantly increasing the risk of heart attack, stroke, kidney failure, and vision loss.

Therefore, blood pressure control is equally important as blood glucose management. Most guidelines recommend that people with diabetes maintain a blood pressure level below 130/80 mmHg, although individual targets may vary. (American Diabetes Association, 2025).

Managing blood pressure also requires making healthy lifestyle choices and taking medication when needed. Reducing salt intake, eating more fruits and vegetables, maintaining a healthy weight, increasing physical activity, and quitting smoking are foundational steps. When these measures are insufficient, medications such as angiotensin-converting enzyme inhibitors (ACEi) or angiotensin receptor blockers (ARBs) are often preferred, as they also protect the kidneys, an organ particularly vulnerable to the effects of diabetes.

High cholesterol and triglycerides are also common in people with type 2 diabetes. Excess cholesterol accelerates the formation of plaque in arteries, contributing to atherosclerosis and elevating the risk of cardiovascular events. For individuals with diabetes, cholesterol targets are stricter. Statins are the most common medications prescribed, but lifestyle changes remain crucial. Replacing saturated fats with healthy fats, increasing fibre intake, maintaining a healthy weight, and engaging in regular exercise all make a significant difference. It is essential to monitor cholesterol levels at least once a year, or more often if medication adjustments are required.

Another important condition linked to diabetes, particularly in women, **is polycystic ovary syndrome (PCOS).** It is characterised by irregular menstrual cycles, elevated levels of androgens (male hormones), and often, cysts on the ovaries. Many women with PCOS experience insulin resistance, which not only increases the risk of developing type 2 diabetes but also complicates blood sugar control. Addressing insulin resistance through a balanced diet, regular exercise, and effective weight management can help improve both blood sugar control and symptoms of **PCOS.** Doctors may also prescribe metformin, a medication commonly used for type 2 diabetes, to help manage both conditions. For women trying to conceive, additional therapies or referrals to a fertility specialist may be necessary.

Chronic kidney disease (CKD) is both a complication of diabetes and a common coexisting condition. The combination of high blood sugar and high blood pressure can damage the small blood vessels in the kidneys, reducing their ability to filter waste from the blood. Regular monitoring of kidney function through blood and urine tests allows for early detection and intervention. Management involves tight control of both blood sugar and blood pressure, as well as dietary adjustments to limit sodium. Furthermore, depending on the disease stage and laboratory findings, adjustments may be made to protein, potassium, and phosphorus intake. Sometimes, medication regimens may need to be adjusted because the kidneys are less effective at clearing certain drugs from the body.

Managing multiple conditions simultaneously requires a holistic, patient-centred approach. This may involve synchronising medication routines, streamlining appointments, and creating a straightforward plan with your healthcare team. Open communication about symptoms, medication side effects, and daily challenges is essential. Importantly, all treatment plans should be personalised;

what works for one individual may not be suitable for another, especially as health circumstances and goals change.

Ageing with Diabetes

Living longer with diabetes presents both challenges and opportunities. As people age, the risk of complications such as heart disease, nerve damage, vision loss, and kidney disease increases. Older adults may also experience more fluctuations in blood sugar levels, sometimes due to changes in kidney function, appetite, or physical activity. Medications that previously worked well may need adjustment, particularly if concerns arise about low blood sugar (hypoglycaemia), memory changes, or difficulty managing complex regimens.

Routine monitoring remains crucial, and treatment goals may change as people age. For example, doctors may recommend slightly higher A1C targets for some older adults to reduce the risk of hypoglycaemia, especially if their life expectancy is limited or they have other serious health issues. Risks of falls, mobility issues, and cognitive health all need attention when planning meals, physical activity, and medication routines.

Social connections become increasingly important with age. Isolation and depression are more common among older adults with chronic disease, and both can negatively impact self-care. Community resources, home care services, and diabetes education programmes can all help maintain independence and quality of life.

Women's Health and Diabetes

Diabetes can affect women's health in distinctive ways throughout their lives. For young women, PCOS, as previously mentioned, not only impacts blood sugar but can also influence fertility, menstrual cycles, and mental health. For those planning a pregnancy, preconception counselling is vital. Maintaining good blood sugar levels before and during pregnancy lowers the risk of complications for both mother and baby. Gestational diabetes, which occurs during pregnancy, increases the risk of developing type 2 diabetes later in life for both mother and child, making regular monitoring and healthy lifestyle choices essential.

Women with diabetes are at a higher risk of developing urinary tract infections and yeast infections due to elevated blood glucose levels, which can promote the growth of bacteria and fungi. Regular gynaecological care and good blood sugar management can help reduce these risks.

Postmenopausal women may notice changes in how their bodies respond to insulin and may need to adjust their diabetes management plan.

Heart disease is sometimes under-recognised in women, yet diabetes increases cardiovascular risk substantially, particularly after menopause. Paying attention to blood pressure, cholesterol, and body weight is just as vital for women as it is for men. Women should know how stress, depression, and life transitions can affect their ability to manage diabetes.

CHAPTER 14
YOUR LONG-TERM WELLNESS PLAN

Diabetes management is a lifelong journey, but it does not have to feel burdensome. Your long-term wellness plan is more than just keeping track of your blood sugar or counting calories; it is also about imagining a life that is full of energy, happiness, and sustainability. The choices you make today will impact your health, energy, and quality of life for years to come, whether you aim to prevent diabetes, manage it, or achieve remission from it.

The first step in making a long-term plan is to be clear about what you want to achieve. It should not just be about numbers on a chart. Think about the life you want to have. How do you want to feel in five, ten, or twenty years? By focusing on things that matter to you, such as being active with your family, travelling without restrictions, or simply having the energy to enjoy life every day, you can discover a motivation that extends beyond any short-term goal.

Long-term wellness begins with making sustainable lifestyle choices. Eating well, staying more active, getting sufficient sleep, and managing stress are not short-term actions; instead, they are lifelong commitments that demand continuous dedication. Consuming balanced, whole-food meals, being mindful of portion sizes, and paying attention to your eating habits can help lower insulin resistance and maintain stable blood sugar levels. Regular exercise, whether it is brisk walking, strength training, or participating in fun sports, supports heart and brain health, enhances overall well-being, and helps regulate blood sugar levels. Managing stress and ensuring adequate sleep are essential. Without sufficient sleep or effective stress management, maintaining healthy habits can become a significant challenge.

Embracing change is a vital part of your long-term wellness plan. Being adaptable is essential, as life is full of surprises. Various factors can influence routines, including work commitments, travel, social occasions, and unexpected stressors. Do not see these as failures but as opportunities to adapt. Prepare for situations that may challenge your habits, such as packing healthy snacks for trips, incorporating exercise into your busy schedule, or utilising stress-reduction techniques during periods of high stress. This method ensures your wellness plan remains practical and achievable.

To stay successful, you need to regularly monitor your progress and reflect on it. Keeping track of your progress through blood glucose readings, weight management, or lifestyle journaling provides you with feedback and fosters greater responsibility. It is essential to think about your journey. Celebrate your achievements and the positive changes you have made. Reflection turns everyday management into a purposeful and empowering process.

Long-term wellness also involves enjoying the good things in life. Diabetes does not mean giving up things; it means making informed choices that are good for your health and overall well-being. Do things you enjoy, eat food that nourishes you, spend time with people you care about, and do hobbies that bring joy and fulfilment. Making wellness a part of your life, rather than viewing it as a set of rules, can help you stay committed to it and maintain a positive outlook for a long time.

Another important factor to consider is preventing complications and maintaining remission. Regular medical check-ups with your healthcare professional, early identification of risk factors, and sticking to your personalised treatment plan can help you stay proactive about your health. Individuals aiming to achieve remission must maintain a healthy weight, remain physically active, and consume a balanced diet. Recognising that remission is a journey, not a one-time event, will help you stay committed while celebrating your progress.

Ultimately, your long-term wellness plan is centred on vision and empowerment. It is about seeing diabetes not as a problem, but as an opportunity to take charge of your health and create the life you want. The decisions you make today about how you eat, move, sleep, and manage stress add up over time and can lead to a future filled with life, energy, and freedom from the problems that many people fear.

To be happy and healthy, whether you have diabetes or not, is all about finding the right balance between caring for your health and enjoying life to the fullest. You can protect your body and enhance your life by adopting a holistic, long-term approach to health. A long-term wellness plan is not a fixed path; it is a living guide that evolves as your needs, circumstances, and goals change over time.

As you progress, remember that every decision you make, from what you eat to how you manage stress, has a lasting impact on your future. These decisions are not about striving for perfection; they are about persevering, learning, and recognising the small victories along the way. They accumulate over time to create a life that is healthier, more energising, and profoundly rewarding.

Ultimately, diabetes does not define who you are. It is just one part of your story, not the whole story. The true measure of success is not only in numbers or tests; it is in the quality of life you create, the joy you nurture, and the strength you develop. You can look forward to a life where health, happiness, and fulfilment go hand in hand if you are intentional, kind to yourself, and consistent in your efforts.

As you adopt these practices and mindset, you embark on a journey where every choice you make not only improves your health but also grants you greater freedom to live fully and authentically.

CONCLUSION AND FINAL WORDS

You Are Not Defined by Your Diagnosis.

It's easy to let a diagnosis like diabetes feel as though it defines you, but remember, you are much more than any number, label, or test result. Diabetes is just one part of your story, not the entire story. You are a person first, a friend, someone with dreams and talents that make you unique. Your diagnosis may influence some of your choices, but it never diminishes your worth or what you can achieve.

Consider this: imagine yourself five years from now, writing a postcard to your present self. Visualise all the successes and experiences that today's choices have made possible and thank yourself for the dedication to health and the resilience to keep moving forward. Let this vision of your future self serve as a reminder, showing you that each step you take today shapes the story you will share tomorrow.

Celebrating Progress, Not Perfection.

Forget about chasing perfection; it is the small steps that matter. Perhaps you swapped soda for water today, took a walk even when you did not feel like it, or made a doctor's appointment you had been putting off. That is progress! Celebrate those wins, no matter how small. Health is a journey, not a finish line. Some days will be more challenging than others, and that is normal. What matters is that you keep showing up, keep learning, and keep moving forward. Be kind to yourself when things do not go as planned. Every effort adds up, and every healthy choice is a victory.

Your health journey is uniquely yours. This book is not the end; it is the beginning of informed, empowered choices. Keep learning, keep asking questions, and keep building a lifestyle that suits you—every small, consistent step counts.

NEXT STEPS

If you are ready for your next step, remember that you do not have to figure everything out on your own.

Consult with your healthcare team, reach out to your local diabetes support groups, or connect with friends and family for additional support. There are excellent resources available, such as apps, community programmes, classes, and even online forums full of people encouraging one another. Take things at your own pace and do not be afraid to ask for help. The journey may twist and turn, but with knowledge, support, and a little self-compassion, you have what it takes to thrive.

Remember, you are resilient, capable, and making progress towards a healthier you. One step at a time and one small change at a time.

FREQUENTLY ASKED QUESTIONS (FAQ)

Q1: How can I tailor the recommendations in this book to suit my specific cultural, dietary, or medical needs?

A: Work with your healthcare teams, such as a dietitian, diabetes specialist team, or your doctor, to tailor advice to your preferences and medical circumstances. You can adapt meal plans to include foods you enjoy, modify recipes for cultural or religious diets, and consider any other health conditions you may have (for example, kidney disease or high blood pressure). Small, realistic changes that fit your lifestyle are more sustainable than strict, one-size-fits-all rules.

Q2: What are the first three steps I should take if I feel overwhelmed by all this information?

A: Track your current habits: Note what you eat, how much you move, and your blood glucose patterns for a few days. Pick one small change, such as adding a 10-minute daily walk or replacing sugary drinks with water. Set a simple, achievable goal: Focus on one goal at a time to build confidence and momentum before tackling additional changes.

Q3: What should I do if I find it hard to stay motivated or encounter setbacks while making lifestyle changes?

A: Setbacks are normal—do not see them as failures. Break goals into smaller steps, celebrate small wins, and keep a journal to track progress. Find strategies that suit your lifestyle, such as pairing exercise with a favourite activity or preparing meals in advance. Professional support (health coach, dietitian, diabetes educator) and peer encouragement can make a significant difference.

Q4: How can I recognise when lifestyle changes are no longer enough, and medication becomes necessary?

A: Your healthcare professional will monitor your blood sugar levels, A1C, and overall health. If your blood glucose levels remain above target despite consistent lifestyle changes, medication may be recommended. Do not see this as a personal failure—type 2 diabetes is progressive, and medications serve as tools to help your body manage blood sugar safely while you maintain healthy habits.

Q5: Where can I find local or online support groups for ongoing encouragement and advice?

A: Local: Ask your clinic, hospital, or diabetes educator about community support groups or classes. Many hospitals run free or low-cost sessions.

Online: Reliable groups include:

- American Diabetes Association (ADA): diabetes.org/community
- Diabetes UK: diabetes.org.uk

REFERENCES:

1. International Diabetes Federation. (2025). Diabetes Atlas. https://diabetesatlas.org/

2. Diabetes is "a pandemic of unprecedented magnitude" now affecting one in 10 adults worldwide. Diabetes Research and Clinical Practice, Volume 181, 109133

3. American Diabetes Association Professional Practice Committee. (2023). 2. Diagnosis and Classification of Diabetes: Standards of Care in Diabetes—2024. Diabetes Care, 47 (Supplement_1), S20–S42.

4. DeMarsilis, A., Reddy, N., Boutari, C., Filippaios, A., Sternthal, E., Katsiki, N., & Mantzoros, C. (2022). Pharmacotherapy of type 2 diabetes: An update and future directions. Metabolism - Clinical and Experimental, 137. https://doi.org/10.1016/j.metabol.2022.155332

5. Lean, M. E., Leslie, W. S., Barnes, A. C., Brosnahan, N., Thom, G., McCombie, L., Kelly, T., Irvine, K., Peters, C., Zhyzhneuskaya, S., Hollingsworth, K. G., Adamson, A. J., Sniehotta, F. F., Mathers, J. C., McIlvenna, Y., Welsh, P., McConnachie, A., McIntosh, A., Sattar, N., & Taylor, R. (2024). 5-year follow-up of the randomised Diabetes Remission Clinical Trial (DiRECT) of continued support for weight loss maintenance in the UK: An extension study. The Lancet Diabetes & Endocrinology, 12(4), 233–246. https://doi.org/10.1016/S2213-8587(23)00385-6

6. Reduction in the Incidence of Type 2 Diabetes with Lifestyle Intervention or Metformin. New England Journal of Medicine, 346(6), 393–403. https://doi.org/10.1056/NEJMoa012512

7. Elbel, B. (2011). Consumer Estimation of Recommended and Actual Calories at Fast Food Restaurants. Obesity (Silver Spring, Md.), 19(10), 1971–1978. https://doi.org/10.1038/oby.2011.214

8. Erbakan, A. N., Arslan Bahadir, M., Gonen, O., & Kaya, F. N. (2024). Mindful Eating and Current Glycemic Control in Patients With Type 2 Diabetes. Cureus, 16(3), e57198. https://doi.org/10.7759/cureus.57198

9. Frontera, W. R., & Ochala, J. (2015). Skeletal muscle: A brief review of structure and function. Calcified Tissue International, 96(3), 183–195. https://doi.org/10.1007/s00223-014-9915-y

10. Thau, L., Gandhi, J., & Sharma, S. (2025). Physiology, Cortisol. In StatPearls. StatPearls Publishing. http://www.ncbi.nlm.nih.gov/books/NBK538239/

11. Luli, M., Yeo, G., Farrell, E., Ogden, J., Parretti, H., Frew, E., Bevan, S., Brown, A., Logue, J., Menon, V., Isack, N., Lean, M., McEwan, C., Gately, P., Williams, S., Astbury, N., Bryant, M., Clare, K., Dimitriadis, G. K., … Miras, A. D. (2023). The implications of defining obesity as a disease: A report from the Association for the Study of Obesity 2021 annual conference. eClinicalMedicine, 58. https://doi.org/10.1016/j.eclinm.2023.101962

12. Clemente-Suárez, V. J., Redondo-Flórez, L., Beltrán-Velasco, A. I., Martín-Rodríguez, A., Martínez-Guardado, I., Navarro-Jiménez, E., Laborde-Cárdenas, C. C., & Tornero-Aguilera, J. F. (2023). The Role of Adipokines in Health and Disease. Biomedicines, 11(5), 1290. https://doi.org/10.3390/biomedicines11051290

13. Ryan, D. H., & Yockey, S. R. (2017). Weight Loss and Improvement in Comorbidity: Differences at 5%, 10%, 15%, and Over. Current Obesity Reports, 6(2), 187–194. https://doi.org/10.1007/s13679-017-0262-y

14. Kim, J. Y., Lee, D. Y., Lee, Y. J., Park, K. J., Kim, K. H., Kim, J. W., & Kim, W.-H. (2015). Chronic alcohol consumption potentiates the development of diabetes through pancreatic β-cell dysfunction. World Journal of Biological Chemistry, 6(1), 1–15. https://doi.org/10.4331/wjbc.v6.i1.1

15. Alcohol and Diabetes | ADA. (n.d.). Retrieved August 14, 2025, from https://diabetes.org/health-wellness/alcohol-and-diabetes

16. Maddatu, J., Anderson-Baucum, E., & Evans-Molina, C. (2017). Smoking and the Risk of Type 2 Diabetes. Translational Research: The Journal of Laboratory and Clinical Medicine, 184, 101–107. https://doi.org/10.1016/j.trsl.2017.02.004

17. England, N.H.S. (n.d.). NHS England» Modifiable risk factors: High impact interventions. Retrieved August 14, 2025, from https://www.england.nhs.uk/ourwork/prevention/secondary-prevention/modifiable-risk-factors-high-impact-interventions/

Other in-text References

- Basterfield, L., Reilly, J. J., Pearce, M. S., & Adamson, A. J. (2022). Changes in children's physical fitness, BMI, and health-related quality of life during the COVID-19 lockdown in the UK. Pediatric Obesity, 17(4), e12855. https://doi.org/10.1111/ijpo.12855

- Hillsdon, M., Rees, T., Ukoumunne, O. C., Metcalf, B., & Solomon, E. (2013). Personal, social, and environmental correlates of physical activity in adults living in rural south-west England: A cross-sectional analysis. International Journal of

Behavioral Nutrition and Physical Activity, 10, 129. https://doi.org/10.1186/1479-5868-10-129

- McCrorie, P., Mitchell, R., Macdonald, L., Jones, A., Coombes, E., Schipperijn, J., & Ellaway, A. (2020). The relationship between living in urban and rural areas of Scotland and children's physical activity and sedentary levels: A country-wide cross-sectional analysis. BMC Public Health, 20, 1–10. https://doi.org/10.1186/s12889-020-8311-y
- Office for Health Improvement and Disparities. (2025). Diabetes profile: Statistical commentary, March 2025. https://www.gov.uk/government/statistics/diabetes-profile-update-march-2025/diabetes-profile-statistical-commentary-march-2025
- Public Health England. (2025). Diabetes profile update: March 2025. https://www.gov.uk/government/statistics/diabetes-profile-update-march-2025
- BMJ Best Practice. (n.d.). Type 1 diabetes – Epidemiology. BMJ. Retrieved September 29, 2025, from https://bestpractice.bmj.com/topics/en-gb/25/epidemiology
- Willett, W. C. (2001). Eat, drink, and be healthy: The Harvard Medical School guide to healthy eating. Free Press.
- Bellamy, L., Casas, J. P., Hingorani, A. D., & Williams, D. (2009). Type 2 diabetes mellitus after gestational diabetes: A systematic review and meta-analysis. The Lancet, 373(9677), 1773–1779. https://doi.org/10.1016/S0140-6736(09)60731-5
- Diabetes UK. (n.d.). Type 2 diabetes. Retrieved from https://www.diabetes.org.uk/about-diabetes/type-2-diabetes
- Diabetes UK. (n.d.). Diabetic nephropathy (kidney disease). Retrieved from https://www.diabetes.org.uk/about-diabetes/looking-after-diabetes/complications/kidneys-nephropathy
- Kidney Research UK. (2024, October 24). Diabetes and kidney disease: how diabetes affects your kidneys. Retrieved from

https://www.kidneyresearchuk.org/conditions-symptoms/diabetes/

- Li, S., Zhao, J. H., Luan, J., Luben, R., Rodwell, S. A., Khaw, K.-T., & Loos, R. J. F. (2011). Genetic predisposition to obesity leads to increased risk of developing type 2 diabetes, which is completely mediated by its obesity-predisposing effect. PLoS ONE, 6(8), e21380. https://doi.org/10.1371/journal.pone.0021380

- McCarthy, M. I. (2001). Susceptibility gene discovery for common metabolic and endocrine traits. Journal of Molecular Medicine, 79(8), 443–451. https://doi.org/10.1007/s001090100236

- NHS. (n.d.). Type 2 diabetes – What is type 2 diabetes? Retrieved from https://www.nhs.uk/conditions/type-2-diabetes/what-is-type-2-diabetes/

- The Diabetes Control and Complications Trial Research Group. (1993). The effect of intensive treatment of diabetes on the development and progression of long-term complications in insulin-dependent diabetes mellitus. New England Journal of Medicine, 329(14), 977–986. https://doi.org/10.1056/NEJM199309303291401

- Ludwig, D. S. (2016). Always hungry?: Conquer cravings, retrain your fat cells, and lose weight permanently. Grand Central Life & Style.

APPENDICES:

1. Websites & National Organisations

1. American Diabetes Association (ADA)

   https://diabetes.org/

2. ADA Professional – Standards of Care

   https://professional.diabetes.org/

3. ADCES (Association of Diabetes Care & Education Specialists)

   https://www.adces.org/

4. Diabetes Food Hub (recipe and meal planning platform)

   https://diabetesfoodhub.org/

5. Diabetes UK

   https://www.diabetes.org.uk/

6. Diabetes Research & Wellness Foundation (UK)

   https://www.drwf.org.uk/

7. NHS – Type 2 Diabetes Support

   https://www.nhs.uk/conditions/type-2-diabetes/support/

8. Diabetes Specialist Nurse Forum (UK) resource hub

   https://www.diabetesspecialistnurseforumuk.co.uk/
   living-with-diabetes

2. Support Groups & Online Communities

1. DiabetesSisters (peer support for women)

   https://diabetessisters.org/

2. Beyond Type 2

   https://beyondtype2.org/

3. TuDiabetes

   https://tudiabetes.org/

4. Diabetes Daily

   https://www.diabetesdaily.com/

5. Defeat Diabetes Foundation

   https://www.verywellhealth.com/diabetes-support-groups-6537603 (listed via Verywell Health overview)

6. Diabetes UK Local Support Groups directory

   https://www.diabetes.org.uk/support-for-you/community-support-and-forums/local-support-groups

7. HealthUnlocked – Diabetes Communities

   https://www.healthunlocked.com/

3. Mobile Apps & Digital Tools

1. mySugr

   https://www.mysugr.com/

2. BlueStar App (via ADCES danatech directory)

   https://www.adces.org/education/danatech/apps-dtx/find-apps-tools

3. Freestyle Libre App

   https://www.freestyle.abbott/us-en/products/freestyle-libre-app.html

4. Diabetes: Recommended Apps from HealthLine

   https://www.healthline.com/health/diabetes/top-iphone-android-apps

5. myDesmond (DESMOND app for type 2)

   https://www.desmond.nhs.uk/

6. myDiabetes (myMhealth platform)

   https://mymhealth.com/mydiabetes

4. Books & Educational Materials

1. Mayo Clinic: The Essential Diabetes Book, 3rd Edition

   https://mcpress.mayoclinic.org/product/mayo-clinic-the-essential-diabetes-book-3rd-edition/

2. Medical Management of Type 2 Diabetes (ADA)

   https://diabetesjournals.org/books/pages/BooksByTitle

3. The Everything Guide to Managing Type 2 Diabetes

   https://www.simonandschuster.com/books/The-Everything-Guide-to-Managing-Type-2-Diabetes/Paula-Ford-Martin/Everything/9781440551963

4. Bright Spots & Landmines (Goodreads listing)

   https://www.goodreads.com/shelf/show/diabetes

5. Mastering Diabetes (Barnes & Noble listing)

   https://www.barnesandnoble.com/b/books/health-diseases-disorders/diabetes/_/N-29Z8q8Z11kc

6. Practical Type 2 Diabetes: A Handbook for Clinicians

   https://shopdiabetes.org/collections/professional-books?srsltid=AfmBOooeXCERGHdofed1twhh9HmMM9iHne5vZl-WaRNTFCc4ZLuq0I6eI